Comprehensive Lifestyle Intervention for Obesity

Tracey Cormier

ABSTRACT

Since 1970 the prevalence rate of adult obesity in the United States (US) has increased dramatically. The Centers for Disease Control and Prevention (CDC) estimate one-third of US adults were overweight (BMI > 25.0 and < 30.0kg/m2) and one-third were obese (BMI ≥ 30.0 kg/m2). Obesity prevalence rates were above 20% in all 50 US states. Obesity-related conditions are serious and can increase the risk of heart disease, stroke, type II diabetes, and some types of cancer. In large part due to these obesity-induced health problems, obesity carries a substantial financial burden, contributing to approximately $147 billion a year in medical costs and is projected to increase by $48-66 billion a year by 2030. There is therefore a considerable health and economic incentive to combat obesity.

Medications, surgery, endoscopic procedures and lifestyle interventions are the main weight loss strategies available to health care providers to manage obesity. There are 5 FDA-approved weight loss drugs that are moderately effective, but quite expensive. Endoscopically placed gastric balloons have been recently approved for weight loss, but they are even more expensive and have to be removed after 6 months. Bariatric surgery remains an alternative for severely obese (BMI > 40 kg/m2) participants who fail less costly and invasive approaches. Comprehensive lifestyle weight management programs provide the foundation for virtually every medical intervention for obesity, even if medications or procedures are indicated. lifestyle interventions provide the cornerstone of obesity management and are prescribed as first-line treatment. Effective comprehensive lifestyle programs use cognitive behavioral interventions to achieve long-term positive changes in physical activity and nutrient intake. There are great variations in the components constituting any given intervention because there is no singular "gold standard" lifestyle intervention.

Currently there are many challenges with lifestyle interventions such as modest weight loss results, sustained weight loss, high dropout rates, and loss of follow up. Current evaluation practices focus exclusively upon end results of weight loss so the reasons behind intervention failures or modest results are not easily discerned. Many times the failures are generically blamed on the programs inability to implement strong behavioral change strategies. However, there are no reliable tools to evaluate the nutrition knowledge component of lifestyle intervention programs.

As part of the Obesity Treatment Research Program (OTRP) in Rochester MN, we collected data on 156 participants. The overall goal of my thesis is to develop and adapt methods that will systematically assess and improve the nutrition education component of a lifestyle intervention

Aim 1:

To describe the methods of establishing a high intensity, year-long, comprehensive lifestyle treatment program for the medical management of obesity at Mayo Clinic, Rochester, MN, that is consistent with the recommendations of the 2013 American College of Cardiology/American Heart Association Task Force on Practice Guidelines and The Obesity Society Guidelines for the Management of Overweight and Obesity in Adults.

Aim 2:

To evaluate outcomes of the Obesity Treatment Research Program to provide a benchmark for subsequent program improvement interventions.

Aim 3:

To develop a novel weight management nutrition knowledge questionnaire that assesses nutrition knowledge as it relates to weight management. The questionnaire will focus on the nutritional dimensions of five key areas: (1) portion size, (2) energy density of foods, (3) reliable nutrition information sources, (4) alcohol and sugar sweetened beverages, (5) variety of food affects intake.

CHAPTER 1

INTRODUCTION

INTRODUCTION

1.1 Obesity background

According to data gathered by the American Heart Association, approximately 78 million United States (US) adults are obese and an additional 76 million are overweight. These numbers are based off cut-offs using the Body Mass Index (BMI), which is calculated from the weight and height of an individual. Obese adults are at high risk for complications of obesity, and those with BMIs from 25 to 29.9 kg/m^2 (overweight) should be considered for screening for metabolic risk[1]. Over the last 30 years, there has been a steady increase in adult BMI; U.S. adult obesity prevalence has more than doubled since the 1960's[2]. The most obvious contributors to this increase are the changes in food consumption[3,4] (i.e. caloric intake, portion distortion, fast food trends, cost of healthy foods, processed foods, etc.) and decreased activity[5,6] (energy expended at work, technological advances, transportation, etc.). Obesity remains one of the top two preventable causes of death[7] and contributes to a host of adverse medical consequences, including heart disease, diabetes, stroke, certain types of cancer, fatty liver disease, and sleep apnea[8].

1.2 Epidemiology of obesity

Obesity rates continue to increase, with approximately 93 million of United States (US) adults affected by the disease. Obesity varies greatly across the US. Arkansas, Alabama, Louisiana, Mississippi, and West Virginia are on the high end with a prevalence rate of 35% or greater. States such as Colorado, the District of Columbia, and Massachusetts have lower prevalence of obesity between 20% and <25% (Figure 1). These numbers also vary by other demographics. For instance, obesity prevalence is approximately 14% in children ages 2-5, 18.5% in youth ages 6-11, and 20.6% in adolescents ages 12-19. The prevalence of obesity is lower in young adults aged 20–39 years and more common in middle-aged and older groups. According to the CDC, individuals with lower income and/or education levels are at higher risk for obesity. Looking at race and ethnicity, African American adults are one and a half times as likely to be obese compared to Caucasian adults. Hispanic or Latino populations also have a higher rate of obesity and are 50% more likely to die from diabetes compared to Caucasians[9] (Figure 2).

1.3 Health disparities and obesity

Although obesity prevalence has increased dramatically, the increase has been greater in low socioeconomic and racial minority groups. Socioeconomic status plays an important role in the wellbeing of our US population. According to the CDC, those with lower income and/or education levels are at greater risk of obesity. Obesity is less common in men and women who have a college degree compared to those with lower education background. The prevalence of obesity is less in adults age 20–39 years and more common in middle-aged and older adults (Figure 2).

Sex analysis reveals that men and women are equally affected by obesity, as there are no significant differences in this disease's prevalence between men and women[9] (Figure 3). Although obesity prevalence for all populations has dramatically increased over the years, higher prevalence rates for low socioeconomic groups and minority groups remains a priority for public health, as socioeconomic status is a key determinant of health and wellbeing in the US population.

Figure 1- 2016 Obesity Prevalence in the United States

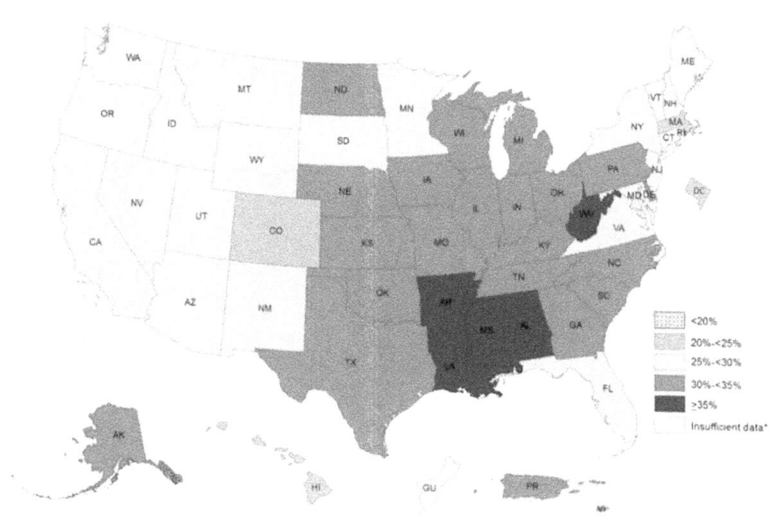

Source: Behavioral Risk Factor Surveillance System, CDC

Figure 2- Prevalence of obesity among adults aged 20 and over, by sex and age: United States, 2015–2016

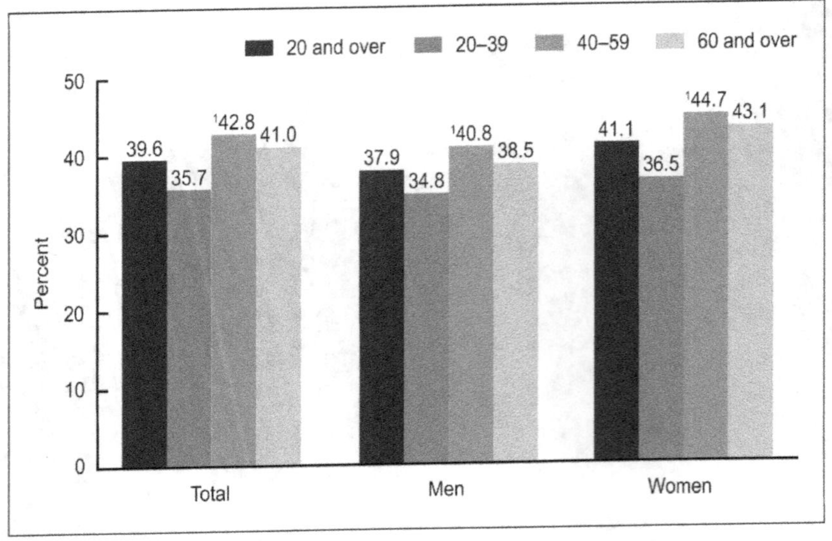

¹Significantly different from those aged 20–39.
NOTES: Estimates for adults aged 20 and over were age adjusted by the direct method to the 2000 U.S. census population using the age groups 20–39, 40–59, and 60 and over. Crude estimates are 39.8% for total, 38.0% for men, and 41.5% for women.

SOURCE: NCHS, National Health and Nutrition Examination Survey, 2015–2016

Figure 3- Age-adjusted prevalence of obesity among adults aged 20 and over, by sex and race and Hispanic origin: United States, 2015–2016

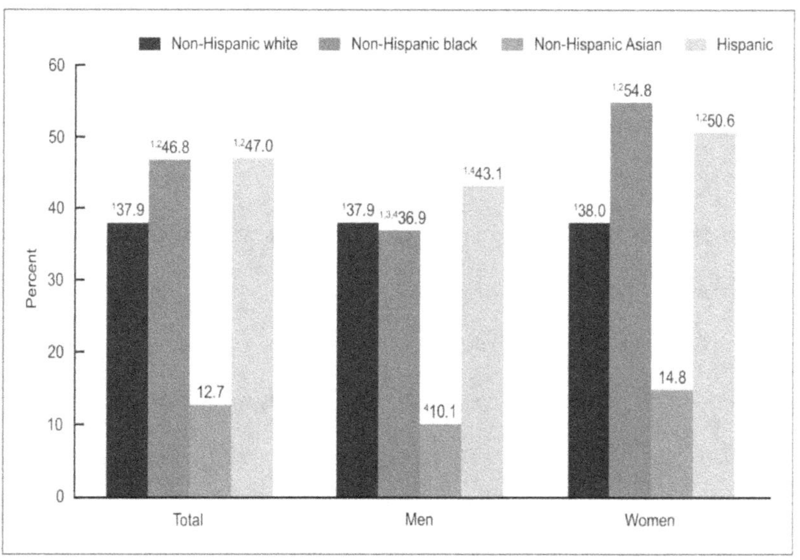

[1]Significantly different from non-Hispanic Asian persons.
[2]Significantly different from non-Hispanic white persons.
[3]Significantly different from Hispanic persons.
[4]Significantly different from women of same race and Hispanic origin.

SOURCE: NCHS, National Health and Nutrition Examination Survey, 2015–2016

1.4 The financial burden of obesity

Obesity imposes a threat to the world's economic burden health. In 2014, approximately two billion people in the globe are suffered from obesity and obesity complications. That is an estimated 30% of the world's population. Obesity also carries a heavy economic burden with both direct medical costs for diagnosis and treatment of disease and indirect costs with value of lost work, insurance, and low wages. Obesity medical costs have increased from an estimated $78.5 billion in 1998 to $147 billion in 2008. Obese adults spend an average of 42% more on direct healthcare costs compared to individuals with a normal BMI; this averages to an additional $1,429 per year[10]. It is estimated that Medicare spending would decrease by 8.5%, and Medicaid spending would be decreased by 11.8% in the hypothetical absence of Obesity. In another study that looked at the 2006 medical spending across all payers; comparison of the obese to healthy-weight individuals showed that spending is 41.5% higher because of obesity[11]. Finally, it is projected that the medical cost of obesity will increase by $48 to $66 billion by 2030[12].

1.5 The medical burden of obesity

The negative effects of obesity on health are varied and well established. The life expectancy is reduced by 6.5 years (BMI of 40-44.9) to 13.7 years (BMI of 55-59.9)[13]. There is well documented evidence that links obesity to an increase the risk of hypertension[14], diabetes mellitus[8,15], coronary artery disease[16], cerebrovascular incident[17], obstructive sleep apnea[18], and deep vein thrombosis[19,20].

1.5.2 Effects of obesity on the cardiovascular system

The decrease in cardiac contractility in obesity has multiple effects downstream. Increases in myocardial thickness result in left ventricular diastolic dysfunction, decreased cardiac compliance, and diastolic heart failure. Concentric hypertrophy of the left ventricle further decreases contractile efficiency. The prevalence of hypertension (HTN) in obese patients is approximately 70%[21]. Systemic hypertension increases left ventricular afterload, increases peripheral resistance, and increases conduit artery stiffness. This can worsen diastolic dysfunction in obesity[22]. Obesity is also associated with increased cholesterol and increased plaque deposition in the coronary arteries, worsening or causing ischemic heart disease. Patients with obesity are more likely to suffer an acute myocardial infarction (MI) compared to patients without obesity[23]. Patients with obesity are also more likely to suffer an MI at a younger age[24].

1.5.2 Relationship between obesity and obstructive sleep apnea

Obese patients can have an increase work of breathing which can increase PaC02 (hypercapnia). This phenomenon is known as obesity hypoventilation syndrome[25].Obesity is also a known risk factor for obstructive sleep apnea because of excessive tissue in the pharynx and tongue. This excessive tissue can result in airway obstruction during sleep. The chronic hypoxia results in hypoxic pulmonary vasoconstriction, which results in pulmonary hypertension. This can led to right ventricular strain, hypertrophy, and eventually heart failure[26].

1.5.3 Metabolic effects of obesity

There are numerous negative ways that obesity can affect the metabolic pathways and paracrine functions. For example, Growth factors, platelet activating factors, cytokines TNF alpha, and IL-6 are proinflammatory cytokines that are related to obesity and linked with atherosclerotic disease. Moreover, high LDL/VLDL levels and abnormal non-HDL to HDL ratios are all risk factors for atherosclerotic disease and are all related to obesity. Hyperuricemia is also more likely in obesity and is associated with cardiovascular disease such as coronary heart disease (CHD), stroke, and hypertension[27,28]. Obesity causes insulin resistance; adult patients with a BMI of 40 or higher have an odds ratio of 7.37 of being diagnosed with diabetes when compared to adults with a normal BMI[29].

1.6 Methods to treat obesity

There are four different, but often complementary approaches used for the medical management of obesity: comprehensive lifestyle modification (diet, activity, and cognitive behavior therapy), pharmaceuticals (Orlistat, Belviq, Qsymia, Saxenda, and Contrave) [30], devices and bariatric surgery. Comprehensive lifestyle interventions are the safest way to lose weight. Comprehensive lifestyle interventions are at the cornerstone of treating obesity[31].

1.6.1 Medications to treat obesity

There are currently five FDA-approved prescription drugs approved for chronic administration to treat obesity (Orlistat, Belviq, Qsymia, Saxenda, and Contrave) and one FDA-approved over-the-counter drug (Alli, which is a lower dose of Orlistat). These weight loss medications have side effects that range from mild (transient nausea, constipation, and diarrhea) to severe (mood disorders up to severe depression and memory loss)[30,32]. Additionally, these drugs can be quite costly because most insurance companies might not coverage weight loss medications[33].

1.6.2 Surgical procedures to treat obesity

Another option for obesity treatment of obesity is bariatric surgery, which is available in restrictive, malabsorptive, or combined approaches[34]. These surgeries can result in immediate postoperative or delayed nutritional complications and thus, surgery is only indicated for participants with BMIs over 40 kg/m^2 who have failed non-surgical treatment or patients with BMIs between 35 and 39.9 kg/m^2 with serious health problems that can be expected to improve with successful weight loss[35] [36].

1.6.3 Endoscopic procedures to treat obesity

There are now multiple endoscopic procedures that are designed to assist in weight management. An endoscopically placed intragastric balloon works by occupying intragastric space and producing early satiety sensation. It can result in up to 15% loss of original body weight. It is approved for six months use in patients with a BMI of 30 to 40 BMI. However, insurance providers in the United States typically do not cover this procedure because of weight regain after the balloon is removed[37]. Other endoscopically preformed procedures included aspiration therapy [38], endoscopic gastric sleeve and endoscopic intragastric injections. There are complications that can occur, and some patients do not qualify for this treatment option.

1.7 Lifestyle interventions in the literature

Although pharmaceuticals, devices and surgery are options for severely obese patients, these treatments require proper diet and physical activity to maintain efficacy. Thus, lifestyle interventions provide the cornerstone of obesity management and are prescribed as first-line treatment[39]. Most insurance companies will cover a few nutrition consults per year, but this is not enough to see clinically meaningful results. A comprehensive lifestyle intervention is administered in group setting which can decrease the cost compared to one on one nutrition consultation sessions.

1.7.1 Nutritional knowledge intervention

The American College of Cardiology/American Heart Association Task Force on Practice Guidelines and The Obesity Society reviewed more than 2000 scholarly articles on Lifestyle interventions[31]. They developed recommendations based on 51 trials (72 articles) that were rated to be of good or fair quality and included all 3 components of life style interventions (dietary prescription, physical activity, and behavioral therapy). Based on these 51 trials they recommended the following:

1-The principal components of an effective high-intensity, on-site comprehensive lifestyle intervention includes a) prescription of a moderately reduced-calorie diet, b) a program of increased physical activity, and c) the use of behavioral strategies to facilitate adherence to diet and activity recommendations.

2-Comprehensive Interventions when compared with usual care produce a weight loss of about 5-10% of the initial weight.

3-Programs should be at least 6 months of high intensity sessions (14 sessions or more in 6 months) to be effective. There is also some evidence that one yearlong programs are superior to six months programs

4-Low- to moderate-intensity lifestyle interventions for weight loss provided to overweight or obese adults by primary care practices alone have not been shown to be effective.

5-Of the overweight/obese adults who participate in a high intensity long-term comprehensive lifestyle intervention, 35% to 60% maintain a loss of ≥5% of initial body weight at ≥2 years[31].

1.7.2 Results of comprehensive life style interventions

Comprehensive lifestyle interventions when compared with usual care produce a weight loss of about 5-10% of the initial weight before comprehensive lifestyle intervention. Lifestyle intervention results remain modest compared to other obesity management approaches. The Look AHEAD trial published in 2007 was a multicentered, randomized, controlled trial lifestyle intervention projects. The study enrolled over 5,000 overweight or obese participants with diabetes. Participants lost an average of 8.6% of their initial body weight[40]. This was one of the largest most successful studies published. A study was conducted by Hollis et al. in 2009 and was published in the American Journal of Preventative Medicine. This was a six months weight loss trial that enrolled 1685 overweight and obese individuals to a 20 weight loss group sessions over the course of six months. The program focused on calorie restriction, moderate-intensity physical activity, and DASH (dietary approaches to stop hypertension). The average participant attended between 14 of the 20 intervention sessions and mean weight loss was 5.8kg[41]. A study by Wadden et al. enrolled 390 participants enrolled in a two-year randomized trial conducted. This study was significant because it was conducted through primary care practices; patients lost 4.6 kg. Of those enrolled, the retention rate was 86% for those who completed the 2-year trial [42]. There are multiple other studies published in the literature describing a lifestyle intervention programs; it is quite evident, however, that most of these studies showed modest weight loss results post intervention.

1.7.3 Challenges in Design and Evaluation of Comprehensive Obesity Lifestyle Interventions

Based on this extensive literature review high intensity life style interventions that include all 3 components are an effective clinical tool for overweight and obese patients. We can also conclude that there is still work that needs to be done to improve the overall effectiveness of these programs. Greater weight loss targets should be the goal because it is clear that the greater the proportion of successful patients and more weight that is lost, the more the benefit. Sustained weight loss of 3%–5% achieved by intervention programs is likely to result in clinically meaningful reductions in triglycerides, blood glucose, hemoglobin A1c (HbA1c), and the risk of developing type 2 diabetes. However, on average it requires even greater weight loss to reduce blood pressure (BP), improve low-density lipoprotein cholesterol (LDL–C) and high-density lipoprotein cholesterol (HDL–C), and reduce the need for medications to control BP, blood glucose, and lipids (10). Therefore, programs should aim to achieve greater weight loss in a larger proportion of enrollees. Another challenge for weight loss programs is helping patients to maintain the weight loss that they have achieved. Only 35% to 60% of the patients are able to maintain their weight loss for over 2 years [31]. When primary outcome is not achieved, or modestly achieved results, it is generically assumed that the behavioral component was lacking, or the patient is not motivated enough. However, the real issue is that no proper tools are available to assess some of the elements of comprehensive life style interventions. For example, when it comes to nutritional knowledge; general nutrition knowledge questionnaires are used to assess knowledge gain[43] because no weight management specific nutritional knowledge questionnaires are available. There are currently no tested tools that can evaluate the learned changes in behavior that aid weight management. Furthermore, a huge challenge is that there is no available tool that predicts dropouts or underachievers in lifestyle interventions. There are some published data about predictors, but it is not enough to make any substantial management decisions prior to offering lifestyle intervention program as treatment option to patients. These are all example of challenges when designing or attempting to improve a lifestyle intervention program.

1.7.4 Mayo Obesity Treatment Research Program (OTRP)-

The Obesity Treatment Research Program is a one-year lifestyle program that focuses on cognitive behavior therapy, nutritional education designed to reduce energy intake, and a physical activity prescription designed to increase activity to a level that will reduce the risk of weight regain. The participants enrolled in this program are largely Olmsted County residents; patients are referred to the program by their primary care provider if they meet the inclusion criteria. They must be adults between the ages of 18-65 and have a BMI between 27-49.9 kg/m^2. Participants are excluded from the study if they have had any previous obesity surgeries. The program includes weekly meetings of a group of 10-20 participants for the first three months, bi-weekly meetings for the following three months, and once a month meeting for the remaining six months. Pre- and post of OTRP measurements include weight BMI, waist, hip, and neck as well as systolic and diastolic blood pressure are conducted. As part of this study, participants allow the investigators to use medical records to assess the long-term outcomes of participation, even if the volunteer does not complete the program. This unique study design allows us to gain follow-up data on a much greater proportion of enrollees than occurs with most obesity treatment programs[44]. At this point we have collected one-year follow up data on 97% of participants and two-year follow up on 83% of participants.

1.8 Nutrition knowledge

1.8.1 General nutritional knowledge

There is clear evidence that most adults have insufficient nutritional knowledge; obese adults systematically underestimate their calorie intake and overestimate their exercise[45]. Recent evidence has shown that administration of a nutritional knowledge curriculum can result in improved disease management outcomes such as decision-making skills and greater reduction in barriers against disease management[46]. Moreover, studies also show that nutrition education can improve metabolic outcomes (fasting blood glucose and HbA1c) in older patients with diabetes[47]. Furthermore, the investigators of a study of an eight-week intervention that was administered to low income mothers who were obese, or overweight found that improvement in nutritional knowledge was associated with greater weight loss[48].

1.8.2 Assessing general nutritional knowledge

There are multiple validated general nutritional knowledge questionnaires. Most of these questionnaires examine general nutrition knowledge and include topics such as cholesterol, saturated/unsaturated fatty acids, vitamins and antioxidants[49-54]. The General Nutrition Knowledge Questionnaire (GNKQ)[51] and the revised GNKQ (GNKQ-R)[52] have been widely used inside and outside of the UK. The GNKQ questionnaires contains wording specific to the population of the UK, which is a potential limitation to generalizing its use in the US. Yorkshire pudding, crisps, and the use of traffic lights system for nutritional labeling are examples of foods and concepts that might hinder its use in the US. Jones et al developed a nutrition knowledge questionnaire in the US that tested concepts regarding the relationship between disease and diet[53]. Feren et al in Norway developed a nutrition knowledge questionnaire that included topics such as meal pattern, food labeling, and the food plate model[54]. Although all four of these questionnaires were well validated, none of them were specific for weight management.

1.8.3 Health disparities in nutritional knowledge

The U.S. population is becoming diverse every day, it is estimated that 30% of the population belongs to a certain racial or ethnic minority group[55,56]. Health disparity and inequality affects many lives in the United States. There are persistent health disparities and these disparities exist across a wide range of diseases. Health disparities exist across many dimensions. There are millions of people who are affected by higher rates of certain diseases and premature death simply because of their race, ethnicity, gender, sexual orientation, age, education level, income, disability status, socioeconomic status, geographic, and immigrant status[57]. A study conducted by Wang et al. in 2012 found that there were racial and ethnic differences in the nutrition-and health-related psychosocial factors scores. These differences included making food choices and awareness of nutrition-related health risks [58]. Minorities in the United States have had a higher incidence and prevalence of diet related chronic diseases and higher mortality rates from these diseases[55]. Health literacy in the literature has been shown to be very important for individual health; low health literacy is associated with poor health outcomes. Having stronger nutrition knowledge is important for individuals trying to manage or lose weight[59]. A study published in 2006 found that approximately one-third of patients had deficits in understanding nutrition labels. The study reported that poor label comprehension was correlated with low-level literacy and numeracy skills[60].

1.8.4 Weight management specific nutritional knowledge

As discussed above, general nutrition knowledge are concepts related to healthy diet and disease prevention and not necessarily related to weight management. When it comes to knowledge pertaining to effective weight management, we focused on five knowledge domains specific to this topic. These five domains are energy density of foods[61,62], portion sizes[4], variety of foods available at a meal[63], alcoholic and sugar sweetened beverages, and reliable information sources[64].

Studies have shown that people consume approximately the same amount of food (volume) daily. Low energy density foods give feelings of fullness; low energy dense foods are high in water and fiber content and contain few calories per gram of food. We know that portion size have expanded over the last 30 years; the size of meals have increased by 69%. Increased portion size is contributing to the rise of obesity in the United States [65]. A study published in 2017 show that 49% of adults consume at least one sugar sweetened beverage per day (average 145 Kcal/day). Excessive consumption of sugar sweetened beverages may contribute to increased energy intake and contribute to the rise of obesity. Living in the digital age, there is a widespread of medical information floating on the internet. This information is often inaccurate and can translate to improper behavior change.15. Having too many varieties of food can contribute to excessive intake. A study conducted by Rolls et al. indicate that volunteers who were offered three food choices versus one consumed ~20% more food[66]. Fundamental understanding of these five concepts is required for subjects pursuing weight loss.

1.9 Significance of the proposed project

My overall goal was to develop and adapt methods that will systematically assess and improve the nutrition education component of a lifestyle intervention. The evidence reviewed by the obesity guideline expert panel clearly indicates that high intensity lifestyle interventions lasting for at least six months are the treatment of choice for overweight and obese adults, based on both safety and efficacy. In aim 1, our goal was to establish a high intensity one-year comprehensive lifestyle intervention for the medical treatment of obesity. The Obesity Treatment Research Program is a multi-specialty project that was established at Mayo Clinic in Rochester, Minnesota. The program enrolled participants who were overweight or obese and was structured in a group setting with 15–20 participants per group. The program included a nutritional intervention designed to reduce energy intake, a physical activity program and a cognitive behavioral approach to increase the likelihood of long-term adherence. We administered a full battery of psychological surveys prior to enrollment designed to help us identify factors that can predict early dropout and insufficient weight loss. The design of this program allowed us to collect weight loss data for dropouts through access to the EMR. There is very little evidence in the literature regarding predictors of who drops out from lifestyle intervention programs and having this follow up data will help us develop programs that cater for a population that will likely achieve sufficient weight loss.

In aim 2, we assessed OTRP existing program to test the hypothesis that "completers" achieve more weight loss when compared to "dropouts." This gave us a solid platform upon which to collect long-term outcomes data. This project is significant and innovative because most programs are not able to collect data for dropouts. However, because most of these participants were seen by care providers in the Mayo Health System, we were able to abstract weight measurements from the Electronic Medical Record (EMR). We were able to successfully collect weight change outcome data in 97% of enrollees at one year and in 83% of enrollees at two years using electronic medical record.

After assessing the efficacy of the program, we developed new tools to assess program outcomes for future comprehensive lifestyle interventions in aim 3. There were no existing tested tools to review and assess these programs (other than weight loss outcomes). We consulted multiple prominent figures with obesity intervention expertise and found no published or unpublished research conducted to assess nutritional knowledge of participants. Moreover, there seems to be a consensus that weight loss specific nutritional knowledge can still be lacking after completion of a program. This led us to my third aim which was to develop and test a nutrition knowledge questionnaire to assess weigh loss specific nutritional knowledge. We applied the developed questionnaire pre and post nutrition education intervention to a cohort of 119 volunteers. We identified knowledge gaps that existed before intervention and gaps that persist despite receiving the intervention. Our goal was to modify the program curriculum to address common knowledge gaps.

To our knowledge, this study was the first of its kind to address nutrition gaps specific to weight management as opposed to general nutritional knowledge. For example, nutritional knowledge curriculums containing information on cholesterol content, saturated versus unsaturated fatty acids, vitamin content, and antioxidant content of food are not directly related to weight loss. These curriculums also tend to lack content in certain areas such as reading food labels, the caloric content of alcoholic beverages or the concept of energy density of food. Our five areas of nutritional knowledge: (1) portion size, (2) energy density of foods, (3) variety of foods, (4) alcohol and sugar sweetened beverages, (5) nutrition information sources provide a well-rounded complete nutritional knowledge curriculum. These five areas provide the basis of our questionnaire and the basis of the curriculum for the nutrition education. This PhD has allowed me to learn in depth about the design of a comprehensive lifestyle program, assess program outcomes using novel approaches and develop and validate a robust nutrition knowledge questionnaire that can assess participant's nutrition regarding weight management.

REFERENCES

1. Go, A.S., *et al.* Executive summary: heart disease and stroke statistics--2014 update: a report from the American Heart Association. *Circulation* **129**, 399-410 (2014).
2. Hruby, A. & Hu, F.B. The Epidemiology of Obesity: A Big Picture. *PharmacoEconomics* **33**, 673-689 (2015).
3. Livingstone, M.B.E. & Pourshahidi, L.K. Portion Size and Obesity. *Advances in Nutrition* **5**, 829-834 (2014).
4. Ledikwe, J.H., Ello-Martin, J.A. & Rolls, B.J. Portion Sizes and the Obesity Epidemic. *The Journal of Nutrition* **135**, 905-909 (2005).
5. Dwyer-Lindgren, L., *et al.* Prevalence of physical activity and obesity in US counties, 2001–2011: a road map for action. *Population Health Metrics* **11**, 7 (2013).
6. Pietilainen, K.H., *et al.* Physical inactivity and obesity: a vicious circle. *Obesity (Silver Spring)* **16**, 409-414 (2008).
7. Mokdad, A.H., Marks, J.S., Stroup, D.F. & Gerberding, J.L. Actual causes of death in the United States, 2000. *Jama* **291**, 1238-1245 (2004).
8. Pi-Sunyer, X. The medical risks of obesity. *Postgraduate medicine* **121**, 21-33 (2009).
9. Hales, C.M., Carroll, M.D., Fryar, C.D. & Ogden, C.L. Prevalence of Obesity Among Adults and Youth: United States, 2015-2016. *NCHS data brief*, 1-8 (2017).
10. Finkelstein, E.A., Trogdon, J.G., Cohen, J.W. & Dietz, W. Annual medical spending attributable to obesity: payer-and service-specific estimates. *Health affairs (Project Hope)* **28**, w822-831 (2009).
11. Hammond, R.A. & Levine, R. The economic impact of obesity in the United States. *Diabetes, metabolic syndrome and obesity : targets and therapy* **3**, 285-295 (2010).
12. Wang, Y.C., McPherson, K., Marsh, T., Gortmaker, S.L. & Brown, M. Health and economic burden of the projected obesity trends in the USA and the UK. *Lancet (London, England)* **378**, 815-825 (2011).
13. Kitahara, C.M., *et al.* Association between class III obesity (BMI of 40-59 kg/m2) and mortality: a pooled analysis of 20 prospective studies. *PLoS medicine* **11**, e1001673 (2014).
14. Jiang, S.Z., Lu, W., Zong, X.F., Ruan, H.Y. & Liu, Y. Obesity and hypertension. *Experimental and therapeutic medicine* **12**, 2395-2399 (2016).
15. Field, A.E., *et al.* Impact of overweight on the risk of developing common chronic diseases during a 10-year period. *Arch Intern Med* **161**, 1581-1586 (2001).
16. Artham, S.M., Lavie, C.J., Milani, R.V. & Ventura, H.O. Obesity and hypertension, heart failure, and coronary heart disease-risk factor, paradox, and recommendations for weight loss. *The Ochsner journal* **9**, 124-132 (2009).
17. Mitchell, A.B., *et al.* Obesity increases risk of ischemic stroke in young adults. *Stroke* **46**, 1690-1692 (2015).
18. Schwartz, A.R., *et al.* Obesity and obstructive sleep apnea: pathogenic mechanisms and therapeutic approaches. *Proceedings of the American Thoracic Society* **5**, 185-192 (2008).
19. Klovaite, J., Benn, M. & Nordestgaard, B.G. Obesity as a causal risk factor for deep venous thrombosis: a Mendelian randomization study. *Journal of internal medicine* **277**, 573-584 (2015).

20.   Yang, G., De Staercke, C. & Hooper, W.C. The effects of obesity on venous thromboembolism: A review. *Open journal of preventive medicine* **2**, 499-509 (2012).

21.   Roche, S.L. & Silversides, C.K. Hypertension, obesity, and coronary artery disease in the survivors of congenital heart disease. *The Canadian journal of cardiology* **29**, 841-848 (2013).

22.   Vasan, R.S. Cardiac function and obesity. *Heart (British Cardiac Society)* **89**, 1127-1129 (2003).

23.   Zhu, J., *et al.* The incidence of acute myocardial infarction in relation to overweight and obesity: a meta-analysis. *Archives of medical science : AMS* **10**, 855-862 (2014).

24.   Basoor, A., *et al.* High prevalence of obesity in young patients with ST elevation myocardial infarction. *The American heart hospital journal* **9**, E37-40 (2011).

25.   Piper, A.J. Obesity hypoventilation syndrome--the big and the breathless. *Sleep medicine reviews* **15**, 79-89 (2011).

26.   Raisinghani, A., Jen, R., Wilson, J. & Malhotra, A. Obstructive Sleep Apnea Effects on the Right Ventricle and Beyond. *The Canadian journal of cardiology* **31**, 821-822 (2015).

27.   Kaur, J. A comprehensive review on metabolic syndrome. *Cardiology research and practice* **2014**, 943162 (2014).

28.   Juraschek, S.P., Miller, E.R., 3rd & Gelber, A.C. Body mass index, obesity, and prevalent gout in the United States in 1988-1994 and 2007-2010. *Arthritis care & research* **65**, 127-132 (2013).

29.   Mokdad, A.H., *et al.* Prevalence of obesity, diabetes, and obesity-related health risk factors, 2001. *Jama* **289**, 76-79 (2003).

30.   Yanovski, S.Z. & Yanovski, J.A. Long-term drug treatment for obesity: a systematic and clinical review. *Jama* **311**, 74-86 (2014).

31.   Jensen, M.D., *et al.* 2013 AHA/ACC/TOS guideline for the management of overweight and obesity in adults: a report of the American College of Cardiology/American Heart Association Task Force on Practice Guidelines and The Obesity Society. *Circulation* **129**, S102-138 (2014).

32.   Christensen, R., Kristensen, P.K., Bartels, E.M., Bliddal, H. & Astrup, A. Efficacy and safety of the weight-loss drug rimonabant: a meta-analysis of randomised trials. *Lancet (London, England)* **370**, 1706-1713 (2007).

33.   Yang, Z. & Hall, A.G. The financial burden of overweight and obesity among elderly Americans: the dynamics of weight, longevity, and health care cost. *Health services research* **43**, 849-868 (2008).

34.   Brethauer, S.A., Chand, B. & Schauer, P.R. Risks and benefits of bariatric surgery: current evidence. *Cleveland Clinic journal of medicine* **73**, 993-1007 (2006).

35.   O'Brien, P.E., *et al.* Treatment of mild to moderate obesity with laparoscopic adjustable gastric banding or an intensive medical program: a randomized trial. *Annals of internal medicine* **144**, 625-633 (2006).

36.   Schauer, P.R., *et al.* Bariatric surgery versus intensive medical therapy for diabetes--3-year outcomes. *N Engl J Med* **370**, 2002-2013 (2014).

37.   Almeghaiseeb, E.S., Ashraf, M.F., Alamro, R.A., Almasoud, A.O. & Alrobayan, A.A. Efficacy of intragastric balloon on weight reduction: Saudi perspective. *World journal of clinical cases* **5**, 140-147 (2017).

38.   Noren, E. & Forssell, H. Aspiration therapy for obesity; a safe and effective treatment. *BMC obesity* **3**, 56 (2016).

39. Goodpaster, B.H., *et al.* Effects of diet and physical activity interventions on weight loss and cardiometabolic risk factors in severely obese adults: a randomized trial. *Jama* **304**, 1795-1802 (2010).

40. Pi-Sunyer, X., *et al.* Reduction in weight and cardiovascular disease risk factors in individuals with type 2 diabetes: one-year results of the look AHEAD trial. *Diabetes Care* **30**, 1374-1383 (2007).

41. Hollis, J.F., *et al.* Weight loss during the intensive intervention phase of the weight-loss maintenance trial. *American journal of preventive medicine* **35**, 118-126 (2008).

42. Wadden, T.A., *et al.* A two-year randomized trial of obesity treatment in primary care practice. *N Engl J Med* **365**, 1969-1979 (2011).

43. Barbosa, L.B., Vasconcelos, S.M., Correia, L.O. & Ferreira, R.C. Nutrition knowledge assessment studies in adults: a systematic review. *Ciencia & saude coletiva* **21**, 449-462 (2016).

44. Mikhail, D.S., *et al.* Methodology of a multispecialty outpatient Obesity Treatment Research Program. *Contemporary clinical trials communications* **10**, 36-41 (2018).

45. Lichtman, S.W., *et al.* Discrepancy between self-reported and actual caloric intake and exercise in obese subjects. *N Engl J Med* **327**, 1893-1898 (1992).

46. Miller, C.K., Edwards, L., Kissling, G. & Sanville, L. Evaluation of a theory-based nutrition intervention for older adults with diabetes mellitus. *J Am Diet Assoc* **102**, 1069-1081 (2002).

47. Miller, C.K., Edwards, L., Kissling, G. & Sanville, L. Nutrition education improves metabolic outcomes among older adults with diabetes mellitus: results from a randomized controlled trial. *Preventive medicine* **34**, 252-259 (2002).

48. Klohe-Lehman, D.M., *et al.* Nutrition knowledge is associated with greater weight loss in obese and overweight low-income mothers. *J Am Diet Assoc* **106**, 65-75; quiz 76-69 (2006).

49. Pellegrini, N., *et al.* Development and validation of a food frequency questionnaire for the assessment of dietary total antioxidant capacity. *J Nutr* **137**, 93-98 (2007).

50. Obayashi, S., Bianchi, L.J. & Song, W.O. Reliability and validity of nutrition knowledge, social-psychological factors, and food label use scales from the 1995 Diet and Health Knowledge Survey. *Journal of nutrition education and behavior* **35**, 83-91 (2003).

51. Parmenter, K. & Wardle, J. Development of a general nutrition knowledge questionnaire for adults. *Eur J Clin Nutr* **53**, 298-308 (1999).

52. Kliemann, N., Wardle, J., Johnson, F. & Croker, H. Reliability and validity of a revised version of the General Nutrition Knowledge Questionnaire. *Eur J Clin Nutr* **70**, 1174-1180 (2016).

53. Jones, A.M., *et al.* Reliability and validity of nutrition knowledge questionnaire for adults. *Journal of nutrition education and behavior* **47**, 69-74 (2015).

54. Feren, A., Torheim, L.E. & Lillegaard, I.T. Development of a nutrition knowledge questionnaire for obese adults. *Food & nutrition research* **55**(2011).

55. Satia, J.A. Diet-related disparities: understanding the problem and accelerating solutions. *J Am Diet Assoc* **109**, 610-615 (2009).

56. Perez, A.D. & Hirschman, C. The Changing Racial and Ethnic Composition of the US Population: Emerging American Identities. *Population and development review* **35**, 1-51 (2009).

57. National Academies of Sciences, E., *et al.* in *Communities in Action: Pathways to Health Equity* (eds. Baciu, A., Negussie, Y., Geller, A. & Weinstein, J.N.) (National Academies Press (US)

58.   Wang, Y. & Chen, X. How much of racial/ethnic disparities in dietary intakes, exercise, and weight status can be explained by nutrition- and health-related psychosocial factors and socioeconomic status among US adults? *J Am Diet Assoc* **111**, 1904-1911 (2011).

59.   Berkman, N.D., Sheridan, S.L., Donahue, K.E., Halpern, D.J. & Crotty, K. Low health literacy and health outcomes: an updated systematic review. *Annals of internal medicine* **155**, 97-107 (2011).

60.   Rothman, R.L., *et al.* Patient understanding of food labels: the role of literacy and numeracy. *American journal of preventive medicine* **31**, 391-398 (2006).

61.   Duncan, K.H., Bacon, J.A. & Weinsier, R.L. The effects of high and low energy density diets on satiety, energy intake, and eating time of obese and nonobese subjects. *The American journal of clinical nutrition* **37**, 763-767 (1983).

62.   Rolls, B.J. The relationship between dietary energy density and energy intake. *Physiology & behavior* **97**, 609-615 (2009).

63.   Rolls, B.J., Van Duijvenvoorde, P.M. & Rowe, E.A. Variety in the diet enhances intake in a meal and contributes to the development of obesity in the rat. *Physiology & behavior* **31**, 21-27 (1983).

64.   Worsley, A. Perceived reliability of sources of health information. *Health Education Research* **4**, 367-376 (1989).

65.   Benton, D. Portion size: what we know and what we need to know. *Critical reviews in food science and nutrition* **55**, 988-1004 (2015).

66.   Rolls, B.J., *et al.* Variety in a meal enhances food intake in man. *Physiology & behavior* **26**, 215-221 (1981).

CHAPTER 2

METHODOLOGY OF A MULTISPECIALTY OUTPATIENT

OBESITY TREATMENT RESEARCH PROGRAM

Dalia S. Mikhail[a], Teresa B. Jensen[b], Todd W. Wade[b], Jane F. Myers[b], Jennifer M. Frank[b], Mark Wieland[c], Don Hensrud[a,] M. Molly McMahon[a], Maria L. Collazo-Clavell[a], Haitham Abu-Lebdeh[a], Kurt A. Kennel[a], Daniel L. Hurley[a], Karen Grothe[d], Michael D. Jensen[a]

[a]Division of Endocrinology, Mayo Clinic, 200 1st St SW, Rochester, MN 55905, USA (mikhail.dalia@mayo.edu, hensrud.donald@mayo.edu, mcmahon.molly@mayo.edu, collazoclavell.maria@mayo.edu, abulebdeh.hs@mayo.edu, kennel.kurt@mayo.edu , hurley.daniel@mayo.edu, jensen@mayo.edu)

[b]Department of Family Medicine, Mayo Clinic, 200 1st St SW, Rochester, MN 55905, USA (jensen.teresa@mayo.edu, wade.todd@mayo.edu, myers.jane@mayo.edu, frank.jennifer2@mayo.edu)

[c]Division of Community Internal Medicine, Mayo Clinic, 200 1st St SW, Rochester, MN 55905, USA (wieland.mark@mayo.edu)

[d]Department of Psychiatry and Psychology, Mayo Clinic, 200 1st St SW, Rochester, MN 55905, USA (grothe.karen@mayo.edu)

Corresponding author: Michael D. Jensen, MD

Endocrine Research Unit

200 1st St SW, Rm 5-194 Joseph

Endocrine Research Unit

Rochester, MN 55905 USA

jensen.mayo.edu

507-255-6515 (office)

507-255-4828 (FAX)

ABSTRACT

Despite the large number of U.S. adults who overweight or obese, few providers have ready access to comprehensive lifestyle interventions, the cornerstone of medical obesity management. Our goal was to establish a research infrastructure embedded in a comprehensive lifestyle intervention treatment for obesity. The Obesity Treatment Research Program (OTRP) is a multi-specialty project at Mayo Clinic in Rochester, Minnesota designed to provide a high intensity, year-long, comprehensive lifestyle obesity treatment. The program includes a nutritional intervention designed to reduce energy intake, a physical activity program and a cognitive behavioral approach to increase the likelihood of long-term adherence. The behavioral intervention template incorporated the Diabetes Prevention Program and the Look AHEAD trial materials. The OTRP is consistent with national recommendations for the management of overweight and obesity in adults, but with embedded features designed to identify patient characteristics that might help predict outcomes, assure long-term follow up and support various research initiatives. Our goal was to develop approaches to understand whether there are patient characteristics that predict treatment outcomes.

Keywords: Obesity, Weight Loss, Intensive Lifestyle Program, Exercise Prescription, Intensive Lifestyle Intervention, Individualized Obesity Treatment

1.1 Introduction

Despite how frequently patients present for adiposity-related health problems, many providers do not have access to an organized obesity treatment program that employs all of the modalities needed to implement a comprehensive lifestyle intervention. The optimal outcomes of weight loss medications, bariatric surgery and endoscopic procedures are attained in conjunction with lifestyle treatment that includes a nutritional intervention designed to reduce energy intake, a physical activity program designed to increase energy expenditure, and a cognitive behavioral approach to increase the likelihood of long-term adherence to dietary changes and greater physical activity [1]. Although there are variations in the components of any given lifestyle intervention, there are reasonable templates for the behavioral components of weight management, including the Diabetes Prevention Program and the Look AHEAD protocol [2,3].

The goal of the Obesity Treatment Research Program (OTRP) is to establish a high intensity, year-long, comprehensive lifestyle treatment program for the medical management of obesity at Mayo Clinic, Rochester, MN, that is consistent with the recommendations of the 2013 American College of Cardiology/American Heart Association Task Force on Practice Guidelines and The Obesity Society Guidelines for the Management of Overweight and Obesity in Adults [4]. As part of the development process we sought to build in features that could help to improve the program outcomes by identifying patient characteristics that might predict successful weight loss or early drop out. If successful, this approach will allow future, selective enrollment of adults most likely to benefit from participating in a comprehensive lifestyle program. The nutritional, physical activity, behavioral and pharmacological approaches were developed by consensus amongst groups of primary care and specialty care providers; ancillary protocols were solicited from subspecialty providers.

We have the following 3 sub-goals: 1) To provide this intervention as a resource to Mayo Clinic investigators who wish to study the effects of non-surgical weight loss on health; 2) To provide support to Mayo Clinic investigators to allow them to gather preliminary data for funding proposals; 3) To serve as a "baseline" program to attract prospective, randomized clinical trials from other sources. This program developed an intensive lifestyle intervention to assist patients in modifying eating habits and increasing physical activity. We also developed a strategy to collect data that supports a number of investigators with an interest in adiposity-related illnesses.

1.1.1 Protocol

Study design

Overview

The goal is to enroll a group of subjects approximately every 3 months. This allows for reasonably rapid participation enrollment and utilization of a closed group format with 15-20 participants per group.

Potential participants attend a group information session and are interviewed by the study coordinator. After signing informed consent, they will obtain clinically indicated pre-treatment laboratory studies if they have not had the requisite laboratory examinations done within the previous 6 months. A number of research measures are included in the protocol (Table 2). These measurements are designed to provide data that may help improve the long-term treatment outcomes and to better understand the prevalence of adiposity-related conditions in this population and their response to weight loss.

In addition to cognitive and behavioral therapy concepts taught in group classes, a nutritional intervention designed to reduce energy intake and a physical activity prescription to increase activity will be incorporated. We include an option for weight management pharmacotherapy if deemed appropriate by the participant's primary care provider in conjunction with a co-investigator physician. At the time this protocol was being developed, only orlistat was approved by the Food and Drug Administration for long-term obesity treatment. The education group classes were designed to be one hour in duration and held 0700-0800 hours (before work), 1200-1300 hours (lunch hour) or 1600-1700 hours (after work). Participants were invited to join the group that best fit their schedule after completion of the entry questionnaires.

Eligibility criteria

Inclusion criteria:

- Adult ages 18-65 years

- Body mass index (BMI) 27-39.9 kg/m^2 (the BMI criteria was modified to include those with a BMI up to 49.9 kg/m^2 based upon a requests from referring providers).

- Able to provide informed consent

- Referred from a primary provider after screening with the PHQ-9 to exclude severe depression.

Exclusion criteria:

- Any active health problem that prevents physical activity

- Previous obesity surgery

- Current participation in a program specifically to lose weight

- Use of weight loss medications within the previous 30 days

- Presence of current nonspecific suicidal thoughts as defined by the PHQ-9 (see below)

- Presence of a clinically significant psychiatric condition (psychosis, bipolar disorder or depression) that is insufficiently controlled to allow participation in the study

- A known history (past 24 months) of substance use disorder

- Women who are currently pregnant or lactating

- A major cardiovascular event within the previous 3 months - including cardiac arrhythmia, congestive heart failure, acute coronary syndrome, stroke, transient ischemic attack or peripheral vascular disease and advice from their primary care physician or cardiologist of major contraindications for exercise

- A known history of any condition or factor that the investigator judges to preclude participation or adherence to the study.

Recruitment

Participants in the study are enrolled primarily from the Mayo Clinic Employee and Community Health (ECH) practice and Olmsted Medical Center primary care clinics, both in located in Rochester, MN. The participants can be referred to the program by their primary care provider or may self-refer with documented permission from their primary care provider.

Informed consent

This protocol was reviewed and approved by the Mayo Clinic Institutional Review Board. All participants provide written, informed consent. Because of the need to assess the long-term outcomes, the consent includes permission for investigators to use Mayo Clinic electronic medical records (EMR) for research specifically related to this program. Participants can withdraw permission by notifying the IRB of their desire to do so.

Potential Outcomes and study measures

Entry and outcome measurements will include weight, BMI [5], blood pressure [5], waist circumference, hip circumference, neck circumference, participant retention and dropout rates. Periodic follow up of vital signs and laboratory test results is done using the Mayo Clinic electronic medical record (EMR), including a review of both dropouts and those that complete the program. Information from the questionnaires and EMR will be used to track changes in laboratory results, sleep and mood for those that remain in the program for one year.

Measurements

A number of research measures are included in the protocol (Table 2). These measurements are designed to provide data that may help improve the long-term treatment outcomes and to better understand the prevalence of adiposity-related conditions in this population and their response to weight loss.

Weight will be measured by calibrated scales as previously described [6]. Waist and hip circumferences will be measured using standardized methods by trained personnel [7]. Neck circumference will be measured using the same tape measure. The Endo-PAT procedure [8,9] (Itamar Medical, Caesarea, Israel) will be completed for the first 100 participants (Table 2).

Body composition will be measured by air displacement plethysmography using the BodPod (Life Measurement Inc, Concord, CA). The device will be calibrated before each test against a standardized cylinder. We will obtain each subject's fat mass and fat free mass based on the following Siri equation: Body Fat = $(4.95/\rho - 4.50) \times 100$.

Physical activity will be monitored by asking each participant to acquire a pedometer or other device.

Self-monitoring of dietary quality will be done by either a smart phone application or manual paper records depending upon the volunteer's access to technology.

Research surveys for psychological phenotyping

After signing informed consent, participants are sent 3 e-mail links unique to their identity to allow them to complete the on-line surveys. Potential volunteers who do not complete the surveys are not considered enrolled in the study and are not invited to participate in the program. The survey data is directly entered into the Scientific Data Management System (SDMS) to facilitate data collection and management. A list of the surveys we selected is provided in Table 1. The types and numbers of surveys include: physical activity readiness [10], eating behavior [11-13] and attitudes [14], sleep quality [15,16], quality of life [17], gastrointestinal symptoms [18,19], personal [20] and family history [21] of alcohol and drug use [22], anxiety [23], stress [24], impulsivity [25], resilience [26] and history of childhood abuse (1 question). Some of the questionnaires contain sensitive or personal questions (Table 1). However, because the data is reviewed collectively rather than individually, we can assure volunteers that their privacy will not be jeopardized. We obtained a Certificate of Confidentiality for this study.

Interventions

The comprehensive lifestyle intervention group meetings are held weekly for the first three months, biweekly for the following three months, and monthly for the last six months. During meetings, food intake diaries may be evaluated and physical activity (pedometer or activity monitor data) may be reviewed

<u>Nutrition intervention approach for weight management:</u>

A tiered nutrition intervention was selected because some patients may have greater success with one approach than another. Figure 1 outlines our tiered approach to nutrition intervention.

The planning group consensus was to base the initial dietary program upon a "volumetrics" approach. Low-energy-dense diets incorporated into weight loss programs encourages reduced energy intake without reducing food volume, helping to minimize the feelings of hunger and food deprivation [27]. The diet includes increased vegetables, legumes and fruits and lesser amounts of energy dense foods. A detailed outline of the nutrition intervention approach follows:

1. Energy density principles: Energy density is defined as the ratio of energy to food volume. This will be explained to participants as amount of calories per volume of food consumed; stressing upon the fact that foods with high fiber and high water content are low energy density foods while foods high in fat and low in water content are high energy density foods. We will emphasize the concepts that a high *volume* of food intake can allow satiety while consuming fewer calories and thus aid weight loss. Participants will be given examples of foods on both ends of the energy density spectrum. They will also be taught how to interpret energy density by looking at food labels and comparing the number of grams and number of calories in one food serving [27].

2. Meal Replacements: Patients who are not successful with weight loss after 3 months of nutrition, activity and behavior interventions may transition to the second nutrition intervention tier – a meal replacement approach. The 3-months' time interval is selected to allow sufficient participation in cognitive behavioral group classes to increase the likelihood of success with the volumetric approach. Meal

replacements have been shown to be an effective weight-loss strategy as most meal replacements are calorie-controlled [28]. If employed, the most common strategy is 1-2 meal replacements per day, with a healthy 3rd meal. This 3rd meal will be recommended as a balanced, nutritious meal with a selection of protein, vegetables, whole-grain starch, and optional calorie controlled additions such as dessert.

<u>Physical Activity Intervention for Weight Management</u>

The weight management protocol emphasizes physical activity as an important element of maintaining a healthy weight and improving overall health. The elements of physical activity addressed for participants in the protocol include:

1. The type of activity – we emphasize walking as the primary recommended activity except when the patient has physical limitations that preclude walking. Second choice activities will be at the discretion of the interventionist and will be designed to approximate the same amount of activity as walking.

2. a) The preferred activity is walking, with monitoring using a pedometer or other device. At the beginning of the intervention, we ask participants to provide their step count data weekly for entry into a database. The eventual recommended goal is 10,000 steps per day. We recommend participants employ their step counting device on a daily basis.

   b) For participants unable to walk due to orthopedic limitations we will ask them to choose an alternative activity, such as bicycling or swimming, and to track the amount of time and intensity of that activity. The targeted amount of activity will be equal to the energy expenditure equivalent of 10,000 steps per day. Adjustments to these goals will be based upon clinical indications as determined by the primary care provider and the interventionist.

3. Achieving goal activity – the approach involves an initial 1-2 weeks of baseline assessment followed by gradual increases to achieve goal amounts of activity. The rate of progression is based upon the participant's tolerance and ability to work greater amounts of activity into their daily routine.

<u>Behavior Protocol</u>

We will include the standard elements of cognitive behavior therapy for weight management – self-monitoring, managing expectations, goal setting, stimulus control, stress reduction, problem solving, social support, cognitive restructuring, and relapse prevention. Self-monitoring is a key component, as frequent, consistent self-monitoring for dietary intake is associated with greater weight loss [29-31] We also focus on motivational enhancement strategies (a patient-centered approach that promotes behavior change through exploring ambivalence in a non-judgmental, but directive manner) throughout the program. We adapted intervention materials from the Diabetes Prevention Program, as well as evidence-based mindfulness modules and strategies to enhance motivation [32-35].

<u>Pharmacotherapy Intervention for Weight Management:</u>

The protocol for weight management intervention includes the option for pharmacotherapy as a treatment for weight loss or weight loss maintenance.

Program goal for implementing pharmacotherapy:

1. Participants will need to complete 6 months of nutrition/behavioral/activity intervention before considering orlistat.
2. If the participant is unsuccessful with weight loss efforts (i.e. losing < 5% body weight within 6 months) orlistat will be considered if the following criteria are met:

BMI > 30 kg/m^2 without metabolic complications and < 5% weight loss or

BMI 27-30 kg/m^2, with metabolic complications and < 5% weight loss.

3. If orlistat is considered, the participant will contact their primary care provider to assure that there will be no contraindications to prescribing the medication (e.g. planned pregnancy, use of cyclosporine, severe liver disease, calcium oxalate kidney stones) and for participants to receive adequate education of potential medication side effects and the use of vitamin supplements.

4. If orlistat is prescribed the participant will have a consultation with the research dietitian to receive dietary instructions on how to minimize side effects during orlistat use.

5. If orlistat is used and there is insufficient weight loss (< 5 % of initial weight) after 3 months, the medication will be stopped.

Participant safety

1. In addition to confirming with the primary care provider any safety contraindications to activity, the participants receive an activity evaluation and education to avoid activity-related injury. Subjects who are Mayo employees or their dependents will be able to use resources at the Mayo Clinic Dan Abraham Healthy Living Center (DAHLC) for their activity evaluation and education. In addition, Mayo patient education resources will be provided to all participants. Participants who are not eligible for DAHLC support will receive counseling and advice from a research dietician.

2. We will provide subjects who cannot or do not wish to use the DAHLC with educational support similar to those available at the DAHLC.

3. The Department of Psychiatry and Psychology reviewed current literature through Google, OVID and PSYCH INFO databases for English language articles and found no evidence that any of the screening questionnaires have been shown to

provoke a state of mind requiring urgent intervention. A variety of terms were used to review the literature (i.e., "impact of psychological assessment," "emotional response to research questionnaires," "impact of psychological research/screening").

Program improvement plan

In order to improve the outcomes from this new program we request direct participant feedback with regards to what aspects were helpful and which were not; in essence forms of focus group. We will also assess whether any of the pre-intervention survey results are predictive of early dropout or success and then, if the findings can be replicated, use those surveys as screening tools for entry of future participants. We plan to eventually incorporate survey research tools to determine whether the concepts we are teaching have been well-learned by the participants and whether better knowledge is associated with better outcomes. Finally, we will continue to monitor the literature for evidence that alternative diet approaches are promising and, if so, implement randomized trials within the overall protocol.

Biostatistical considerations

All analyses will be performed utilizing two-sided tests with a significance level α of 0.05. Relevant p-values and 95% confidence intervals (CI) will be reported. Univariate analyses will be reported as proportions and mean where appropriate, accompanied by standard deviations. Multivariate analyses will be performed to control for confounders. Demographic characteristics of participants will be expressed as means plus and minus standard deviation. Average weight loss will be expressed as percentage of original body weight change and 95% CI. Means will be compared between "completers" and "drop outs." Student t tests will be used to compare means and calculated p-values. Odds ratios will be used to assess the likelihood of a psychological assessment tool to predict drop outs. The means of different physiological indices will be compared between completers and dropouts with P values calculated. Because this is not a randomized, prospective trial the statistical analyses will be required to employ adjustments for multiple post-hoc comparisons when testing for associations. The primary prospective hypothesis is that participants who drop out of the program will not lose as much weight as participants who do not drop out. The weight loss for participants who drop out will be obtained from medical record review.

2.1 Discussion

Our comprehensive lifestyle intervention for weight loss is in line with the American College of Cardiology/American Heart Association Task Force on Practice Guidelines and The Obesity Society [4]. The task force recommends that the principal components of an effective high-intensity, on-site comprehensive lifestyle intervention include: a) prescription of a moderately reduced-calorie diet, b) a program of increased physical activity, and c) the use of behavioral strategies to facilitate adherence to diet and activity recommendations. It is also recommended that programs have at least 6 months of high intensity sessions (14 sessions or more in 6 months) to be effective [4]. There is also evidence that one year programs are superior to 6 month programs. In addition, low- to moderate-intensity lifestyle interventions for weight loss provided to overweight or obese adults by primary care practices alone have not been shown to be effective [4,36]. The Obesity Treatment Research Program at the Mayo Clinic, Rochester, Minnesota will provide a unique research model for a high intensity, comprehensive lifestyle treatment program for the medical management of obesity. The research protocol is developed to yield information that will provide for more focused interventions to future participant groups based on evidence from the preceding groups. Specialists in Endocrinology, Sleep

Medicine, Gastroenterology, Cardiology, Psychology and Primary Care Internal Medicine and Family Medicine will participate and collect data from the participants. The protocol includes the ability to enroll up to 500 participants over 5 years.

We suggest that this protocol is unique in several aspects. First, the design allows for the development of a program that acts as a backbone for additional research assessments that are incorporated both at the beginning and later as the program evolves. Second, we employ a comprehensive group of surveys before enrollment that allow us to develop psychological, eating behavior, social, sleep and gastrointestinal phenotyping data that may serve to identify factors that can predict early dropout, poor weight loss or extreme success. The use of a web linked survey result entry system will significantly reduce data entry work load, reduce cost, decrease risk of mistaken entries, and enable us to import metrics directly to electronic data sheets ready for statistical analysis [37]. Another unique aspect of this protocol is that we will collect weight loss data for drop outs through access to the EMR. There is very little research in the literature regarding predictors of who drops out from lifestyle intervention programs [38-40]. This aspect of the protocol will enable us to understand treatment results for both completers and drop outs for extended periods of time as data suggests that 80% of Olmsted County residents are seen at least once in the health care system within one year [41].

This program is initiated with funding support from the Mayo Clinic Rochester Department of Medicine as one of their research efforts. In this way, the initial participants will not have to pay for the services. The goal is to refine and improve the program in order to be able to document success, thereby allowing it to serve as a contract program for research studies sponsored by industry, NIH and professional societies, as well as to attract clinical referrals from insurance providers or patients who are willing to pay out-of-pocket.

3.1 Conclusion

Although there are many different options for the treatment of obesity, there has been little study as to how to select the one(s) most appropriate for an individual patient. Our comprehensive lifestyle program protocol was developed using a multispecialty approach with the goal of collecting data that will allow modification of the program and the different arms to test hypotheses based on review of outcomes. This can lead to stepwise iterations and improvements in long term outcomes based upon the comprehensive intake and follow up data. This is a consensus driven protocol developed by both specialists and primary care providers, and therefore includes multiple research aspects.

4.1 Acknowledgments

This work was supported by the Mayo Clinic Rochester, Minnesota Department of Internal Medicine. This research did not receive any specific grant from funding agencies in the public, commercial, or not-for-profit sectors.

5.1 References

[1] Wadden TA, Webb VL, Moran CH, et al. Lifestyle modification for obesity: new developments in diet, physical activity, and behavior therapy. Circulation. Mar 6 2012;125(9):1157-1170.

[2] The Diabetes Prevention Program (DPP): description of lifestyle intervention. Diabetes Care. Dec 2002;25(12):2165-2171.

[3] Wadden TA, West DS, Delahanty L, et al. The Look AHEAD study: a description of the lifestyle intervention and the evidence supporting it. Obesity (Silver Spring). May 2006;14(5):737-752.

[4] Jensen MD, Ryan DH, Apovian CM, et al. 2013 AHA/ACC/TOS guideline for the management of overweight and obesity in adults: a report of the American College of Cardiology/American Heart Association Task Force on Practice Guidelines and The Obesity Society. Circulation. 2014;129(25 Suppl 2):S102-S138.

[5] Franz MJ, Boucher JL, Rutten-Ramos S, et al. Lifestyle weight-loss intervention outcomes in overweight and obese adults with type 2 diabetes: a systematic review and meta-analysis of randomized clinical trials. Journal of the Academy of Nutrition and Dietetics. Sep 2015;115(9):1447-1463.

[6] Anthanont P, Jensen MD. Does basal metabolic rate predict weight gain? Am J Clin Nutr. Aug 31 2016;104:959-963.

[7] Carranza Leon BG, Jensen MD, Hartman JJ, et al. Self-Measured vs professionally measured waist circumference. Ann Fam Med. May 2016;14(3):262-266.

[8] Kuvin JT, Mammen A, Mooney P, et al. Assessment of peripheral vascular endothelial function in the ambulatory setting. Vascular medicine (London, England). Feb 2007;12(1):13-16.

[9] Axtell AL, Gomari FA, Cooke JP. Assessing endothelial vasodilator function with the Endo-PAT 2000. Journal of visualized experiments : JoVE. Oct 15 2010(44).

[10] Thomas S, Reading J, Shephard RJ. Revision of the Physical Activity Readiness Questionnaire (PAR-Q). Canadian journal of sport sciences = Journal canadien des sciences du sport. Dec 1992;17(4):338-345.

[11] Gearhardt AN, Corbin WR, Brownell KD. Preliminary validation of the Yale Food Addiction Scale. Appetite. Apr 2009;52(2):430-436.

[12] Stunkard AJ, Messick S. The three-factor eating questionnaire to measure dietary restraint, disinhibition and hunger. Journal of psychosomatic research. 1985;29(1):71-83.

[13] Allison KC, Lundgren JD, O'Reardon JP, et al. The Night Eating Questionnaire (NEQ): psychometric properties of a measure of severity of the Night Eating Syndrome. Eating behaviors. Jan 2008;9(1):62-72.

[14] Rieder S, Ruderman A. The development and validation of the weight management support inventory. Eating behaviors. Jan 2007;8(1):39-47.

[15] Buysse DJ, Reynolds CF, 3rd, Monk TH, et al. The Pittsburgh Sleep Quality Index: a new instrument for psychiatric practice and research. Psychiatry research. May 1989;28(2):193-213.

[16] Fritsche L, Greenhalgh T, Falck-Ytter Y, et al. Do short courses in evidence based medicine improve knowledge and skills? Validation of Berlin questionnaire and before and after study of courses in evidence based medicine. BMJ. Dec 7 2002;325(7376):1338-1341.

[17] Pettit T, Livingston G, Manela M, et al. Validation and normative data of health status measures in older people: the Islington study. International journal of geriatric psychiatry. Nov 2001;16(11):1061-1070.

[18] Vakil N, Bjorck K, Denison H, et al. Validation of the reflux symptom questionnaire electronic diary in partial responders to proton pump inhibitor therapy. Clinical and translational gastroenterology. Jan 26 2012;3:e7.

[19] Kulich KR, A. M, Pacini F, et al. Reliability and validity of the Gastrointestinal Symptom Rating Scale (GSRS) and Quality of Life in Reflux and Dyspepsia (QOLRAD) questionnaire in dyspepsia: a six-country study. Health and quality of life outcomes. Jan 31 2008;6:12.

[20] Bohn MJ, Babor TF, Kranzler HR. The Alcohol Use Disorders Identification Test (AUDIT): validation of a screening instrument for use in medical settings. Journal of studies on alcohol. Jul 1995;56(4):423-432.

[21] Mann RE, Sobell LC, Sobell MB, et al. Reliability of a family tree questionnaire for assessing family history of alcohol problems. Drug and alcohol dependence. May 1985;15(1-2):61-67.

[22] Smith PC, Schmidt SM, Allensworth-Davies D, et al. A single-question screening test for drug use in primary care. Arch Intern Med. Jul 12 2010;170(13):1155-1160.

[23] Spitzer RL, Kroenke K, Williams JB, et al. A brief measure for assessing generalized anxiety disorder: the GAD-7. Arch Intern Med. May 22 2006;166(10):1092-1097.

[24] Cohen S, Kamarck T, Mermelstein R. A global measure of perceived stress. Journal of health and social behavior. Dec 1983;24(4):385-396.

[25] Patton JH, Stanford MS, Barratt ES. Factor structure of the Barratt impulsiveness scale. Journal of clinical psychology. Nov 1995;51(6):768-774.

[26] Connor KM, Davidson JR. Development of a new resilience scale: the Connor-Davidson Resilience Scale (CD-RISC). Depression and anxiety. 2003;18(2):76-82.

[27] Rolls BJ, Drewnowski A, Ledikwe JH. Changing the energy density of the diet as a strategy for weight management. J Am Diet Assoc. May 2005;105(5 Suppl 1):S98-S103.

[28] Heymsfield SB, van Mierlo CA, van der Knaap HC, et al. Weight management using a meal replacement strategy: meta and pooling analysis from six studies. Int J Obes Relat Metab Disord. May 2003;27(5):537-549.

[29] Burke LE, Wang J, Sevick MA. Self-monitoring in weight loss: a systematic review of the literature. J Am Diet Assoc. Jan 2011;111(1):92-102.

[30] Laitner MH, Minski SA, Perri MG. The role of self-monitoring in the maintenance of weight loss success. Eating behaviors. Apr 2016;21:193-197.

[31] Peterson ND, Middleton KR, Nackers LM, et al. Dietary self-monitoring and long-term success with weight management. Obesity (Silver Spring). Sep 2014;22(9):1962-1967.

[32] West DS, Gorin AA, Subak LL, et al. A motivation-focused weight loss maintenance program is an effective alternative to a skill-based approach. Int J Obes (Lond). Feb 2011;35(2):259-269.

[33] Mathieu J. What should you know about mindful and intuitive eating? J Am Diet Assoc. Dec 2009;109(12):1982-1987.

[34] Bush HE, Rossy L, Mintz LB, et al. Eat for life: a work site feasibility study of a novel mindfulness-based intuitive eating intervention. American journal of health promotion : AJHP. Jul-Aug 2014;28(6):380-388.

[35] Doll HA, Petersen SE, Stewart-Brown SL. Obesity and physical and emotional well-being: associations between body mass index, chronic illness, and the physical and mental components of the SF-36 questionnaire. Obes Res. Mar 2000;8(2):160-170.

[36] Wadden TA, Volger S, Sarwer DB, et al. A two-year randomized trial of obesity treatment in primary care practice. N Engl J Med. Nov 24 2011;365(21):1969-1979.

[37] Cooper CJ, Cooper SP, del Junco DJ, et al. Web-based data collection: detailed methods of a questionnaire and data gathering tool. Epidemiologic perspectives & innovations : EP+I. Jan 4 2006;3:1.

[38] Roumen C, Feskens EJ, Corpeleijn E, et al. Predictors of lifestyle intervention outcome and dropout: the SLIM study. Eur J Clin Nutr. Oct 2011;65(10):1141-1147.

[39] Bautista-Castano I, Molina-Cabrillana J, Montoya-Alonso JA, et al. Variables predictive of adherence to diet and physical activity recommendations in the treatment of obesity and overweight, in a group of Spanish subjects. Int J Obes Relat Metab Disord. May 2004;28(5):697-705.

[40] Moroshko I, Brennan L, O'Brien P. Predictors of dropout in weight loss interventions: a systematic review of the literature. Obes Rev. Nov 2011;12(11):912-934.

[41] St Sauver JL, Grossardt BR, Yawn BP, et al. Data resource profile: the Rochester Epidemiology Project (REP) medical records-linkage system. Int J Epidemiol. Dec 2012;41(6):1614-1624.

<u>Table 1.</u> Required questionnaires

	Baseline	24 weeks	48 weeks
1.Yale Food Addiction Scale (YFAS) *	X	X	X
2.Barratt Impulsiveness Scale (BIS) *	X		X
3.Family/personal history of addiction *	X		X
4.Alcohol Use Disorders Test (AUDIT) *	X		X
5.Drug use	X		X
6.Childhood Trauma (1 question) *	X		X
7.Self-efficacy for eating	X	X	X
8.Self-efficacy for physical activity *	X	X	X
9.Binge Eating *	X	X	X
10.Generalized Anxiety Disorder (GAD-7) *	X	X	X
11.Perceived Stress Scale (PSS) *	X	X	X
12.CD Resilience Scale (CD-RISC 10) *	X		X
13.Weight Management Support Inventory (WMSI) *	X		X
14.Health Survey Questionnaire (HSQ) *			X
15.European Quality of Life-5 (EQoL-5D) *			X
16. Physical Activity Readiness Q (PAR-Q) *	X		X
17.The Three Factor Eating Questionnaire (TFEQ-R18v2) *	X	X	X
18.Pittsburgh Sleep Quality Index (PSQI) *	X		X
19.Night Eating Questionnaire (NEQ) *	X		X
20.Berlin Questionnaire *	X		X
21.Reflux Symptom Questionnaire (RSQ) *	X	X	X
22.Gastrointestinal Symptom Rating Scale (GSRS) *	X	X	X

<u>Table 2. Program Schedule</u>

Weeks	-2	-1	0	4	8	12	16	20	24	28	32	36	40	44	48
Phone Pre-Screen for study criteria	X														
Informed consent		X													
Medical History	X														
Height		X													
Blood Pressure (BP)		X	X			X			X			X			X
Weight			X	X	X	X	X	X	X	X	X	X	X	X	X
BMI			X	X	X	X	X	X	X	X	X	X	X	X	X
Circumferences - waist, hip and neck			X			X			X			X			X
Fasting blood glucose			X												X
Serum total, HDL and LDL-cholesterol			X												X
Serum triglycerides			X												X
Serum Alanine Transaminase (ALT)			X												X
Serum Aspartate Aminotransferase (AST)															
Stool samples			X			X									X
Endo-PAT			X						X						X

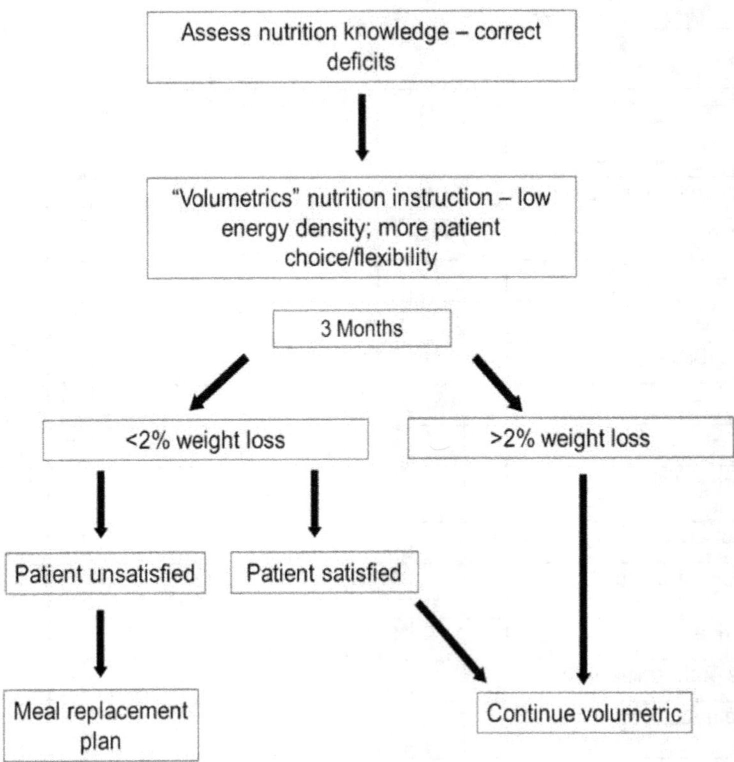

<u>Figure 1.</u> Nutrition Intervention Approach for Weight Management

CHAPTER 3

LONG-TERM IMPACT OF THE OBESITY TREATMENT RESEARCH PROGRAM ON WEIGHT AND CLINICAL OUTCOMES

ABSTRACT

Background:

Obesity can increase the risk for heart disease, stroke, diabetes, hypertension and sleep apnea. Comprehensive lifestyle interventions are the cornerstone for medical management of obesity weight management. Obesity guidelines recommends at least six months intervention that focuses on cognitive behavioral therapy, physical activity, and nutrition education.

Objectives:

To assess outcomes of the Obesity Treatment Research Program (OTRP) at Mayo Clinic after completion or dropout from a six month or a one year comprehensive weight loss intervention. And to analyze one and two year follow up data using Electronic Medical Record (EMR).

Methods:

156 patients, age 18-65, BMI 27-49, in the Olmsted County Employee Community Health practice enrolled prior to May, 2014 and provided written, informed consent allowing electronic medical records (EMR) use to collect follow-up data. Patients were enrolled in the OTRP and received cognitive behavior therapy, nutrition and physical activity education. Eight groups were eligible for data analysis. The same experienced interventionist led each of intervention sessions (>20 in total). Weight was recorded regularly at group sessions and via the EMR for those with <10 months of participation.

Results:

Of the 156 participants enrolled in the program, 113 completed the lifestyle intervention; retention rate was 72%. The overall weight reduction for completers and dropouts was 3.8%.; p-value < 0.00011. Of those subjects, 38% lost at least 5% of their original body weight and about 17% lost at least 10%. We collected weight loss data for 97% of participants at one year and 83% at two years. Waist circumference reduction was 3.4% (p-value <0.00041) and hip circumference reduction was 1.9 cm; p-value < 0.0082 (1.6% reduction) at the one year mark.

Conclusion:

The use of IRB approved consent to track weight loss in dropouts via the EMR allowed us to collect follow-up data on 97% of participants at one year and 83% at two years. This quantitative analysis will inform efforts to improve outcomes and retention.

INTRODUCTION

According to the CDC, more than 35% of the US population is obese and more than 30% are overweight[1]. There are three contributing factors to the rise in obesity in the United States: consumption of high energy dense foods, an excess of energy intake over expenditure, and a decline in physical activity[2-4]. The medical care costs of obesity increased dramatically in the last 30 years. In 2014 obesity contributed to a huge global economic financial burden, the average cost of obesity was approximately $2.0 trillion[5]. Obesity contributes to a high chronic disease burden, and an increased risk of diabetes, stroke, myocardial infraction, sleep apnea[6-8], as well as dramatically reducing life expectancy[9]. Weight loss among overweight and obese individuals is an important target for improving overall health. Weight reduction of 3%-5% of original body weight can result in clinically significant health benefits such as improvement in glycemic control, reduction in blood pressure and triglycerides[10].

There are three different treatment tactics for the medical management of obesity: bariatric surgery, pharmaceutical, and lifestyle interventions[11]. Although surgical procedures and weight loss medications are an effective strategy for weight loss, they may not be an ideal approach for a large percentage of overweight and obese individuals. It is estimated that approximately 1% of severely obese patients undergo a weight loss surgery procedure[12]. There are many complications that can occur from weight loss surgery and some patients do not qualify for this treatment option[13,14]. There are currently several weight loss medications but all have the potential for side effects[15]. However, Surgery and medication treatment options are costly[16-18]. Thus, lifestyle interventions are proposed as first-line treatment therapies for treating obesity. Lifestyle interventions are non-surgical methods that use cognitive behavioral interventions to achieve long-term positive changes in physical activity and nutrient intake[19]. A successful program focuses on decreasing caloric intake, increase physical activity and behavioral therapy modifications. Comprehensive lifestyle interventions have few side effects or complications and are cost-effective compared to surgery and weight loss medications[20]. However, it is unclear why lifestyle interventions are not as effective with only modest weight loss and why weight loss is not uniform across different programs in the US. There are many challenges with current lifestyle interventions such as modest weight loss results, sustained weight loss, high dropout rates and loss of follow up[10].

Previous studies using lifestyle interventions for weight loss in adults with severe obesity showed increased weight loss when compared to minimal or standard care, especially studies using combined diet and exercise components. Improved results have also been shown in programs that last at least six months (i.e., ≥14 sessions in 6 months) in either an individual or group setting led by an experienced interventionist. The 2013 obesity guidelines recommend that a lifestyle intervention program should implement a nutrition knowledge curriculum that focuses on decreasing caloric intake to 1,200–1,500 kcal/day for women and 1,500–1,800 kcal/day for men with focused efforts on teaching participants to restrict high energy dense foods, reduce portion size, and increase fiber rich foods[10].

The goal of this study was to assess the effectiveness of the Obesity Treatment Research Program at Mayo clinic (OTRP). We assessed the weight loss results at one year and two years using Mayo Clinic electronic medical records. The OTRP is a one-year long program that focuses on behavioral weight loss intervention, a curriculum that focuses on increasing physical activity and a curriculum that teaches participants about nutrition knowledge specifically regarding weight management. The OTRP aligns with the obesity guidelines. The study outlines the process of developing and analyzing the OTRP and focusing effort on improving the efficiency and efficacy of this program[21]. We assessed the effectiveness of the OTPR on weight loss as well as program adherence in overweight or obese subjects to improve future program efficiency and efficacy.

METHODS

Methods of this study was describes in chapter 2 of this this dissertation and published in the "Methodology of a multispecialty outpatient Obesity Treatment Research Program[21]." All analyses were performed utilizing two-sided tests with a significance level α of 0.05. Relevant p-values and 95% confidence intervals (CI) was reported. The weight loss for participants who dropped out was obtained from medical record review. The EMR data were accessed through the Unified Data Platform (UDP); the platform is a massive repository where EMR data is replicated into. Access to the platform was granted to research team members through safeguards that require members to provide an IRB number to verify the need for access. An Application Programming Interface (API), maintained by Mayo clinic IT, utilizes a statistical software interface to import data into SAS. Statistical analysis was then performed on the imported data.

RESULTS

One hundred and fifty-six participants were studied; groups 1-7 were enrolled in a one year program and group 8 were enrolled in a six month program. Groups 1-8 had 14-31 participants per group (table 1). Baseline characteristics of participants are demonstrated in table 2; overall, 126 participants were female and 30 participants were male. The mean age was 49.5 years, the mean weight 99.2 kg, and mean BMI 35.2 kg/m2.

Approximately 44% were classified as class I obese 30<=BMI<35 kg/m2, 33.3% Class II Obesity 35<=BMI<40 kg/m2, and 11.5% with severe Obesity BMI>=40 kg/m2. The participants for this study were predominately Caucasian (97%), employed (91%), and had some college or higher degree (89%). There were statistically significant differences between age between groups 1-7 and group 8.

Comorbidity data were collected pre-enrollment using survey methodology and was documented as a "yes or no" by each subject in every group (Table 3). The survey asked participants if they were suffering from the following comorbidities: heart disease, heart failure, lung disease, mobility, obstructive sleep apnea, eating disorders, depression, anxiety, diabetes, and hypertension. The most common comorbid conditions were depression (29.5%), anxiety (13.5%), hypertension (8.3%), and diabetes (7.7%).

The major focus for the analysis was changes in biometrics pre and post-intervention. After enrollment and intervention, participants lost on average 3.8% of their original body weight. Approximately 38% of participants who completed the one year program lost at least 5% of their original body weight and about 17% lost at least 10% of their original body weight. When looking at the two-year results for the completers of the original one year program, only 0.9% reduction in original body weight was noted, this was not statistically significant. Participants on average lost one point in their BMI scale at one year. At the two-year mark, approximately 27% of participants had lost at least 5% of their original body weight and approximately 6% of participants had at least a 10% reduction in weight (table 4). One year data was collected for 151 subjects; we were able to collect weight loss data for 97% of participants at one year and 83% at two years.

The biometrics collected (waist, hip and neck circumference) at one year were not as robust as weight loss data collected and we were able to collect data for only 65-75 participants. There was a statistically significant reduction in waist circumference of approximately four centimeters post intervention. Waist circumference reduction at one year estimated to be 3.4% (p-value <0.00041). Hip circumference was reduced by an average of 1.9 cm; p-value < 0.0082 (1.6% reduction) at the one year mark. Finally, neck circumference reduction was not statistically significant at the one year mark. There was a reduction in both systolic and diastolic blood pressure; however, the degree of reduction was not sufficient to achieve statistical significance (Table 5).

Of the 156 participants, 113 completed the program with a retention rate of 72%. 137 of the 156 patient completed the 1year program (19 were enrolled in group 8 and only had a 6 month program), these were included in the analysis comparing dropouts and completers. Participants who completed a one-year long program lost on average of 3.8% of original body weight. Those who dropped out lost an average of 2.2% of original body weight. However, the difference was not large enough to achieve statistical significance. Among completers vs. dropouts at one year, there was a statistically significant difference between the percentages of participants who were able to achieve at least 5% of weight loss; approximately 38% of completers and 14% of dropouts lost at least 5% of original body weight. The difference at the two-year mark was not statistically significant (table 6). Participants who enrolled in a one year program lost approximately 3.8% of original body weight and participants who enrolled in a six months program lost an average of 0.9% of original body weight when measured at the one year mark p-value= 0.0802. The difference in weight loss between both groups was not enough to achieve statistical significance. Also, 38% of participants from groups 1-7 lost at least 5% of their original body weight while participants from group 8 lost only 16% of their original body weight (Table 7). The difference was close to achieving statistical significant (p=0.0608).

There was no statistically significant difference in participants' ability to lose weight based on their starting BMI. There was also no statistical difference in the percentage of participants that were able to achieve 5% or 10% reduction in their original body weight based on their starting BMI. This was also true when looking at the two-year results; there was no difference in participants' ability to maintain weight loss at two years regardless of their starting BMI (Table 8). Of the participants who lost at least 10% of their original body weight at one year, participants with class II obesity were able to sustain weight loss for two years when compared to participants that were overweight, class I, or class III obese (p=0.0163).

1.4 Discussion

The Obesity Treatment Research Program at the Mayo Clinic, Rochester, Minnesota was developed as a multispecialty outpatient treatment program for overweight and obese outpatients. The OTRP was patterned on the current <u>Guidelines (2013) for Managing Overweight and Obesity</u>[10] for lifestyle/behavioral intervention prior to other treatments for excess weight. Our program had 8 groups of outpatients who attended either a 6 or 12 month program for a total of 156 participants (126 female and 30 male) with a retention rate of 72%. The analysis utilized initial informed consent to access current and future medical records through the EMR. This paper looked at information available at one and two years after enrollment for completers as well as dropouts. The overall average weight reduction for completers and dropouts from original body weight was 3.8%; p-value < 0.00011 using the available records of 97% of the enrollees at one year and 83% at two years. A total of 38% lost at least 5% of their original body weight and 16.5% lost at least 10% of their original body weight. Completers of the one year program (groups 1-7) lost an average of 3.8% of their original body weight and the dropouts lost on average 2.2%; p value= 0.1727.

Access to the patient records through the EMR was invaluable in analyzing the effectiveness of the OTRP. Use of the EMR allowed us to look at features of the program to see if any patient characteristics or outcomes predicted how best to individualize the interventions in future programs. The ability to track participant's long term beyond the program allows us to ascertain any common features that might predict outcomes. Typically, follow up data for as much as 97% of participants is not seen in lifestyle intervention programs. A study conducted by Saaristo et al. reported follow up results for 70.3% of participants in a lifestyle intervention program[22]. This highlights the unique advantage of the OTRP at Mayo Clinic.

There was no statistically significant difference in blood pressure measurements pre and post lifestyle intervention program; this can be attributed to multiple factors. Even though hypertension is expected to improve following weight loss intervention[23], the magnitude of reduction in blood pressure might have not been enough to show a statistically significant difference. Blood pressure measurements are routinely obtained in the primary care office. If measurements are out of normal range, patients are likely to be offered a dose adjustment of their anti-hypertensive medication. This was not controlled for when collecting blood pressure data points and could potentially blunt blood pressure alterations caused by weight changes.

There seemed to be a greater reduction in percentage of body weight lost in participants who completed the intervention when compared to dropouts. However, the difference was not large enough to achieve statistical significance. Investigators had similar challenges comparing weight loss in completers versus dropouts[24]. Not achieving a statistically significant result was probably because the study was originally powered to include 500 participants. Due to lack of funding, a total of 156 individuals were included in the analysis. There was statistically significant difference in the percentage of participants that were able to achieve at least 5% or 10% loss of baseline weight (Table 6). These results indicate the importance of completing the one year lifestyle intervention as opposed to dropping out before the competition of the program. When comparing the amount of weight loss achieved by participants of different obesity classes, it was evident that there were no significant differences in achieving weight loss between the different classes of obesity. Similar findings were reported by Gotthelf et al. when comparing weight loss efficacy by severity of obesity[25]. This confirms that patients regardless of their obesity class are able to benefit from lifestyle intervention programs.

Weaknesses of this study arose from our inability to track all the outcome data form the EMR. Participants who were not followed by the Mayo Clinic for health care did not have subsequent EMR notes or vital signs. Weight and blood pressure are routinely recorded following clinic visits; however, hip, waist and neck circumference measurements are not routinely obtained. We also did not record why patients decided to dropout of the program. This information would have been helpful in our analysis and goal of identifying individual characteristics that could improve the program's outcomes and retention.

CONCLUSION

The Obesity Treatment Research Program at the Mayo Clinic has yielded important information that continues to be analyzed by multiple specialties. The weight loss outcomes have been modest yet positive. Utilization of the EMR system to collect weight loss measurements has proven to be invaluable.

REFERENCES

1. Go, A.S., *et al.* Executive summary: heart disease and stroke statistics--2014 update: a report from the American Heart Association. *Circulation* **129**, 399-410 (2014).
2. McAllister, E.J., *et al.* Ten putative contributors to the obesity epidemic. *Critical reviews in food science and nutrition* **49**, 868-913 (2009).
3. Romieu, I., *et al.* Energy balance and obesity: what are the main drivers? *Cancer causes & control : CCC* **28**, 247-258 (2017).
4. Hill, J.O., Wyatt, H.R. & Peters, J.C. Energy balance and obesity. *Circulation* **126**, 126-132 (2012).
5. Tremmel, M., Gerdtham, U.G., Nilsson, P.M. & Saha, S. Economic Burden of Obesity: A Systematic Literature Review. *International journal of environmental research and public health* **14**(2017).
6. Pi-Sunyer, X. The medical risks of obesity. *Postgraduate medicine* **121**, 21-33 (2009).
7. Jean-Louis, G., Zizi, F., Clark, L.T., Brown, C.D. & McFarlane, S.I. Obstructive sleep apnea and cardiovascular disease: role of the metabolic syndrome and its components. *Journal of clinical sleep medicine : JCSM : official publication of the American Academy of Sleep Medicine* **4**, 261-272 (2008).
8. Jiang, S.Z., Lu, W., Zong, X.F., Ruan, H.Y. & Liu, Y. Obesity and hypertension. *Experimental and therapeutic medicine* **12**, 2395-2399 (2016).
9. Kitahara, C.M., *et al.* Association between class III obesity (BMI of 40-59 kg/m2) and mortality: a pooled analysis of 20 prospective studies. *PLoS medicine* **11**, e1001673 (2014).
10. Jensen, M.D., *et al.* 2013 AHA/ACC/TOS guideline for the management of overweight and obesity in adults: a report of the American College of Cardiology/American Heart Association Task Force on Practice Guidelines and The Obesity Society. *Circulation* **129**, S102-138 (2014).
11. Yanovski, S.Z. & Yanovski, J.A. Long-term drug treatment for obesity: a systematic and clinical review. *Jama* **311**, 74-86 (2014).
12. Sugerman, H.J., Wolfe, L.G., Sica, D.A. & Clore, J.N. Diabetes and hypertension in severe obesity and effects of gastric bypass-induced weight loss. *Annals of surgery* **237**, 751-756; discussion 757-758 (2003).
13. O'Brien, P.E., *et al.* Treatment of mild to moderate obesity with laparoscopic adjustable gastric banding or an intensive medical program: a randomized trial. *Annals of internal medicine* **144**, 625-633 (2006).
14. Ma, I.T. & Madura, J.A., 2nd. Gastrointestinal Complications After Bariatric Surgery. *Gastroenterology & hepatology* **11**, 526-535 (2015).
15. Ioannides-Demos, L.L., Proietto, J., Tonkin, A.M. & McNeil, J.J. Safety of Drug Therapies Used for Weight Loss and Treatment of Obesity. *Drug Safety* **29**, 277-302 (2006).
16. Flum, D.R., *et al.* The use, safety and cost of bariatric surgery before and after Medicare's national coverage decision. *Annals of surgery* **254**, 860-865 (2011).
17. Kwon, S., *et al.* The impact of accreditation on safety and cost of bariatric surgery. *Surgery for obesity and related diseases : official journal of the American Society for Bariatric Surgery* **9**, 617-622 (2013).

18.   Encinosa, W.E., Bernard, D.M., Steiner, C.A. & Chen, C.C. Use and costs of bariatric surgery and prescription weight-loss medications. *Health affairs (Project Hope)* **24**, 1039-1046 (2005).

19.   Lv, N., *et al.* Behavioral lifestyle interventions for moderate and severe obesity: A systematic review. *Preventive medicine* **100**, 180-193 (2017).

20.   Jacobs-van der Bruggen, M.A., *et al.* Lifestyle interventions are cost-effective in people with different levels of diabetes risk: results from a modeling study. *Diabetes Care* **30**, 128-134 (2007).

21.   Mikhail, D.S., *et al.* Methodology of a multispecialty outpatient Obesity Treatment Research Program. *Contemporary clinical trials communications* **10**, 36-41 (2018).

22.   Saaristo, T., *et al.* Lifestyle intervention for prevention of type 2 diabetes in primary health care: one-year follow-up of the Finnish National Diabetes Prevention Program (FIN-D2D). *Diabetes Care* **33**, 2146-2151 (2010).

23.   Neter, J.E., Stam, B.E., Kok, F.J., Grobbee, D.E. & Geleijnse, J.M. Influence of weight reduction on blood pressure: a meta-analysis of randomized controlled trials. *Hypertension (Dallas, Tex. : 1979)* **42**, 878-884 (2003).

24.   Holzapfel, C., *et al.* The challenge of a 2-year follow-up after intervention for weight loss in primary care. *Int J Obes (Lond)* **38**, 806-811 (2014).

25.   Gotthelf, L., *et al.* High intensity lifestyle intervention and long-term impact on weight and clinical outcomes. *PloS one* **13**, e0195794 (2018).

Table 1- Percentage of enrollment per group

Groups	Participants (n and %)
1	17 (10.9%)
2	14 (9.0%)
3	18(11.5%)
4	31 (19.9%)
5	23 (14.7%)
6	17 (10.9)
7	17 (10.9)
8	19 (12.2%)

Table 2: Socio-demographic characteristics of subjects

	Patient Characteristics by Group			
	Group 1-7 (N=137)	Group 8 (N=19)	Total (N=156)	p value
Dropouts				0.22031
Completers	97 (70.8%)	16 (84.2%)	113 (72.4%)	
Dropout	40 (29.2%)	3 (15.8%)	43 (27.6%)	
Baseline Weight				0.65292
N	137	19	156	
Mean	99.5	97.2	99.2	
Height cm				0.77602
N	137	19	156	
Mean	167.9	167.8	167.9	
Baseline BMI				0.25512
N	137	19	156	
Mean	35.2	34.5	35.2	
Severity of Obesity				0.16441
Overweight BMI<30	14 (10.2%)	3 (15.8%)	17 (10.9%)	
Class I Obesity 30<=BMI<35	58 (42.3%)	11 (57.9%)	69 (44.2%)	
Class II Obesity 35<=BMI<40	50 (36.5%)	2 (10.5%)	52 (33.3%)	
Severe Obesity BMI>=40	15 (10.9%)	3 (15.8%)	18 (11.5%)	
Age				0.01172
N	137	19	156	
Mean	50.3	43.9	49.5	
Sex				0.82981
Women	111 (81.0%)	15 (78.9%)	126 (80.8%)	
Men	26 (19.0%)	4 (21.1%)	30 (19.2%)	
Race				0.88311
B	1 (0.7%)	0 (0.0%)	1 (0.6%)	
C	129 (94.2%)	19 (100.0%)	148 (94.9%)	
N	1 (0.7%)	0 (0.0%)	1 (0.6%)	
O	5 (3.6%)	0 (0.0%)	5 (3.2%)	
U	1 (0.7%)	0 (0.0%)	1 (0.6%)	
Education				0.87561
Missing	19	3	22	
High School or GED	7 (5.9%)	0 (0.0%)	7 (5.2%)	
Some College	43 (36.1%)	4 (25.0%)	47 (34.8%)	
Undergraduate	28 (23.5%)	5 (31.3%)	33 (24.4%)	

Patient Characteristics by Group

	Group 1-7 (N=137)	Group 8 (N=19)	Total (N=156)	p value
4 year	8 (6.7%)	1 (6.3%)	9 (6.6%)	
Graduate	32 (26.9%)	6 (37.5%)	38 (28.1%)	
Employment				0.54061
Missing	1	0	1	
No	13 (9.6%)	1 (5.3%)	14 (9.0%)	
Yes	123 (90.4%)	18 (94.7%)	141 (91.0%)	
Marital Status				0.06261
Divorced	6 (4.4%)	0 (0.0%)	6 (3.8%)	
Married	118 (86.1%)	14 (73.7%)	132 (84.6%)	
P	1 (0.7%)	0 (0.0%)	1 (0.6%)	
Single	9 (6.6%)	5 (26.3%)	14 (9.0%)	
Widowed	3 (2.2%)	0 (0.0%)	3 (1.9%)	

[1]Chi-Square
[2]Kruskal Wallis

Table 3- Comorbidity of subjects per group

	Patient Characteristics by Group			
	Group 1-7 (N=137)	Group 8 (N=19)	Total (N=156)	p value
Dx Heart Disease				0.3134[1]
No	130 (94.9%)	19 (100.0%)	149 (95.5%)	
Yes	7 (5.1%)	0 (0.0%)	7 (4.5%)	
Dx Heart Failure				
No	137 (100.0%)	19 (100.0%)	156 (100.0%)	
Dx Lung Disease				0.7087[1]
No	136 (99.3%)	19 (100.0%)	155 (99.4%)	
Yes	1 (0.7%)	0 (0.0%)	1 (0.6%)	
Dx Mobility				0.7087[1]
No	136 (99.3%)	19 (100.0%)	155 (99.4%)	
Yes	1 (0.7%)	0 (0.0%)	1 (0.6%)	
Dx OSA				0.2498[1]
No	128 (93.4%)	19 (100.0%)	147 (94.2%)	
Yes	9 (6.6%)	0 (0.0%)	9 (5.8%)	
Dx Eat				0.0071[1]
No	137 (100.0%)	18 (94.7%)	155 (99.4%)	
Yes	0 (0.0%)	1 (5.3%)	1 (0.6%)	
Dx Depression				0.1980[1]
No	99 (72.3%)	11 (57.9%)	110 (70.5%)	
Yes	38 (27.7%)	8 (42.1%)	46 (29.5%)	
Dx Anxiety				0.6892[1]
No	118 (86.1%)	17 (89.5%)	135 (86.5%)	
Yes	19 (13.9%)	2 (10.5%)	21 (13.5%)	
Dx Addiction				0.7087[1]
No	136 (99.3%)	19 (100.0%)	155 (99.4%)	
Yes	1 (0.7%)	0 (0.0%)	1 (0.6%)	
Diabetes				0.6208[1]
No	127 (92.7%)	17 (89.5%)	144 (92.3%)	
Yes	10 (7.3%)	2 (10.5%)	12 (7.7%)	
Hypertension				0.7121[1]
No	126 (92.0%)	17 (89.5%)	143 (91.7%)	
Yes	11 (8.0%)	2 (10.5%)	13 (8.3%)	

[1]Chi-Square
[2]Kruskal Wallis

Table 4- One year and two year follow up weight loss data

	Total (N=97)	p value
Weight Loss For Subjects Completing The Study		
Baseline Weight		
N	97	
Mean	99.0	
Change in Weight: Year 1 Minus Baseline		<0.0001[1]
N	97	
Mean	-3.7	
% Change in Weight: Baseline to Year 1		<0.0001[1]
N	97	
Mean	-3.8	
Year 1:Lost at Least 5% of Baseline Weight		
No	60 (61.9%)	
Yes	37 (38.1%)	
Year 1:Lost at Least 10% of Baseline Weight		
No	81 (83.5%)	
Yes	16 (16.5%)	
Change in Weight: Year 2 Minus Baseline		0.3077[1]
N	79	
Mean	-0.9	
% Change in Weight: Baseline to Year 2		0.2764[1]
N	79	
Mean	-0.9	
Year 2: Lost at Least 5% of Baseline Weight		
Missing	18	
No	58 (73.4%)	
Yes	21 (26.6%)	
Year 2:Lost at Least 10% of Baseline Weight		
Missing	18	
No	74 (93.7%)	
Yes	5 (6.3%)	

[1]Sign Rank (Mu0=0)

Change in Biometric Parameters Overall		
	Total	p value
Waist cm Baseline		
N	127	
Mean	108.5	
Change in Waist cm: Month 12 Minus Baseline		0.0002[1]
N	66	
Mean	-3.9	
% Change in Waist cm: Month 12 Minus Baseline		0.0004[1]
N	66	
Mean	-3.4	
Hip cm Baseline		
N	124	
Mean	120.3	
Change in Hip cm: Month 12 Minus Baseline		0.0082[1]
N	65	
Mean	-1.9	
% Change in Hip cm: Month 12 Minus Baseline		0.0083[1]
N	65	
Mean	-1.6	
Neck cm Baseline		
N	122	
Mean	38.3	
Change in Neck cm: Month 12 Minus Baseline		0.0856[1]
N	65	
Mean	-0.4	
% Change in Neck cm: Month 12 Minus Baseline		0.1202[1]
N	65	
Mean	-1.0	
Systolic BP Baseline		
N	117	
Mean	126.0	
Change in Systolic BP: Month 12 Minus Baseline		0.6808[1]
N	75	
Mean	-0.2	
% Change in Systolic BP: Month 12 Minus Baseline		0.8294[1]
N	75	
Mean	0.5	
Diastolic BP Baseline		
N	117	
Mean	76.5	
Change in Diastolic BP: Month 12 Minus Baseline		0.1854[1]
N	75	
Mean	1.8	

Change in Biometric Parameters Overall

	Total	p value
% Change in Diastolic BP: Month 12 Minus Baseline		0.1328[1]
N	75	
Mean	3.3	

[1]Sign Rank (Mu0=0)

Table 6- Weight loss results for completers and dropouts

Weight Loss By Study Completion Status				
	Did Not Drop Out (N=97)	Drop Out (N=40)	Total (N=137*)	p value
Baseline Weight				0.4689[1]
N	97	40	137	
Mean	99.0	100.6	99.5	
Change in Weight: Year 1 Minus Baseline				0.2169[1]
N	97	35	132	
Mean	-3.7	-2.2	-3.3	
% Change in Weight: Baseline to Year 1				0.1727[1]
N	97	35	132	
Mean	-3.8	-2.2	-3.4	
Year 1:Lost at Least 5% of Baseline Weight				0.0094[2]
Missing	0	5	5	
No	60 (61.9%)	30 (85.7%)	90 (68.2%)	
Yes	37 (38.1%)	5 (14.3%)	42 (31.8%)	
Year 1:Lost at Least 10% of Baseline Weight				0.0389[2]
Missing	0	5	5	
No	81 (83.5%)	34 (97.1%)	115 (87.1%)	
Yes	16 (16.5%)	1 (2.9%)	17 (12.9%)	
Change in Weight: Year 2 Minus Baseline				0.0990[1]
N	79	35	114	
Mean	-0.9	0.0	-0.6	
% Change in Weight: Baseline to Year 2				0.0941[1]
N	79	35	114	
Mean	-0.9	0.1	-0.6	
Year 2:Lost at Least 5% of Baseline Weight				0.1489[2]
Missing	18	5	23	
No	58 (73.4%)	30 (85.7%)	88 (77.2%)	
Yes	21 (26.6%)	5 (14.3%)	26 (22.8%)	
Year 2:Lost at Least 10% of Baseline Weight				0.3517[2]
Missing	18	5	23	
No	74 (93.7%)	31 (88.6%)	105 (92.1%)	
Yes	5 (6.3%)	4 (11.4%)	9 (7.9%)	

*Excluding group 8 from analysis
[1]Kruskal Wallis
[2]Chi-Square

Table 7- Weight loss results by groups

	Weight Loss By Groups			
	Group 1-7 (N=97)	Group 8 (N=19)	Total (N=116*)	p value
Baseline Weight				0.7484[1]
N	97	19	116	
Mean	99.0	97.2	98.7	
Change in Weight: Year 1 Minus Baseline				0.0802[1]
N	97	19	116	
Mean	-3.7	-1.0	-3.3	
% Change in Weight: Baseline to Year 1				0.0734[1]
N	97	19	116	
Mean	-3.8	-0.9	-3.4	
Year 1:Lost at Least 5% of Baseline Weight				0.0608[2]
No	60 (61.9%)	16 (84.2%)	76 (65.5%)	
Yes	37 (38.1%)	3 (15.8%)	40 (34.5%)	
Year 1:Lost at Least 10% of Baseline Weight				0.0566[2]
No	81 (83.5%)	19 (100.0%)	100 (86.2%)	
Yes	16 (16.5%)	0 (0.0%)	16 (13.8%)	
Change in Weight: Year 2 Minus Baseline				0.8346[1]
N	79	16	95	
Mean	-0.9	-1.3	-1.0	
% Change in Weight: Baseline to Year 2				0.7503[1]
N	79	16	95	
Mean	-0.9	-1.7	-1.1	
Year 2:Lost at Least 5% of Baseline Weight				0.8957[2]
Missing	18	3	21	
No	58 (73.4%)	12 (75.0%)	70 (73.7%)	
Yes	21 (26.6%)	4 (25.0%)	25 (26.3%)	
Year 2:Lost at Least 10% of Baseline Weight				0.1028[2]
Missing	18	3	21	
No	74 (93.7%)	13 (81.3%)	87 (91.6%)	
Yes	5 (6.3%)	3 (18.8%)	8 (8.4%)	

*Excluding dropouts from analysis
1Kruskal Wallis
2Chi-Square

Table 8- Weight reduction by severity of obesity

	Weight Loss By Severity of Obesity					
	Overweight BMI<30 (N=10)	Class I Obesity 30<=BMI<35 (N=44)	Class II Obesity 35<=BMI<40 (N=34)	Severe Obesity BMI>=40 (N=9)	Total (N=97*)	p value
Baseline Weight						<0.0001[1]
N	10	44	34	9	97	
Mean	81.4	95.3	102.2	124.4	99.0	
% Change in Weight: Baseline to Year 1						0.4438[1]
N	10	44	34	9	97	
Mean	-4.4	-4.1	-4.1	-1.0	-3.8	
Year 1:Lost at Least 5% of Baseline Weight						0.8151[2]
No	7 (70.0%)	28 (63.6%)	19 (55.9%)	6 (66.7%)	60 (61.9%)	
Yes	3 (30.0%)	16 (36.4%)	15 (44.1%)	3 (33.3%)	37 (38.1%)	
Year 1:Lost at Least 10% of Baseline Weight						0.6586[2]
No	7 (70.0%)	37 (84.1%)	29 (85.3%)	8 (88.9%)	81 (83.5%)	
Yes	3 (30.0%)	7 (15.9%)	5 (14.7%)	1 (11.1%)	16 (16.5%)	
% Change in Weight: Baseline to Year 2						0.3122[1]
N	8	35	27	9	79	
Mean	-0.6	-0.1	-3.2	2.4	-0.9	
Year 2:Lost at Least 5% of Baseline Weight						0.4804[2]
Missing	2	9	7	0	18	
No	5 (62.5%)	27 (77.1%)	18 (66.7%)	8 (88.9%)	58 (73.4%)	
Yes	3 (37.5%)	8 (22.9%)	9 (33.3%)	1 (11.1%)	21 (26.6%)	
Year 2:Lost at Least 10% of Baseline Weight						0.0163[2]
Missing	2	9	7	0	18	
No	8 (100.0%)	35 (100.0%)	22 (81.5%)	9 (100.0%)	74 (93.7%)	
Yes	0 (0.0%)	0 (0.0%)	5 (18.5%)	0 (0.0%)	5 (6.3%)	

*Excluding dropouts and group 8
[1]Kruskal Wallis
[2]Chi-Square

CHAPTER 4
DEVELOPMENT AND VALIDATION TESTING OF A WEIGHT MANAGEMENT NUTRITION KNOWLEDGE QUESTIONNAIRE FOR ADULTS

Mikhail, Dalia S[1], Rolls, Barbara J[2], Yost, Kathleen J[3], Balls-Berry, Joyce E[4], Gall, Margaret M[5], Blixt, Kristen R[5], Novotny, Paul J, Albertie[6], Monica L[7], Jensen, Michael D[1].

[1]Endocrine Research Unit, Mayo Clinic, Rochester, Minnesota, USA

[2]Department of Nutritional Sciences, The Pennsylvania State University, University Park, PA, USA

[3]Health Science Research, Mayo Clinic, Rochester, MN, USA

[4]Department of Health Sciences Research, Division of Epidemiology, Center for Clinical and Translational Science Community Engagement Program, Mayo Clinic, Rochester, Minnesota, USA

[5]Clinical Nutrition, Mayo Clinic, Rochester, Minnesota, USA

[6]Department of Biomedical Statistics and Informatics, Mayo Clinic, Rochester, Minnesota, USA

[7]Office of Health Disparities Research, Mayo Clinic, Jacksonville, Florida, USA

Keywords: energy density, portion size, food variety, sugar sweetened beverages

Running title: Development and testing of the WMNKQ

Correspondence: Michael D. Jensen, M.D.

Mayo Clinic, Endocrine Research Unit

200 1st Street SW, Rm 5-194 Joseph, Mayo Clinic

Rochester, MN 55905 USA

Phone: +1 507 255-6515

Fax: +1 507 255-4828

E-mail: jensen.michael@mayo.edu

Funding: Supported by grants DK40484, DK45343 and CTSA Grant Number UL1 TR002377 from the National Center for Advancing Translational Sciences (NCATS), a component of the National Institutes of Health (NIH). The content is solely the responsibility of the authors and does not necessarily represent the official views of the NIH.

Disclosure: The authors declared no conflict of interest.

Author Contributions: DM – designed and performed the studies, analyzed the data, and wrote the manuscript. MG, KB and MA performed the studies, reviewed and edited the manuscript. BR, KY and J B-B designed the study and edited the manuscript. PN analyzed the data and edited the manuscript. M.D.J. designed, performed and oversaw the study, reviewed and edited the manuscript.

Study Importance Questions

- Increased knowledge of the topic is needed for appropriate behavior change

- There is no validated questionnaire that addresses the topics of food properties specific to weight management

- The Weight Management Nutrition Knowledge Questionnaire met accepted psychometric requirements for such an instrument and should prove useful in understanding the role of nutrition knowledge in weight management.

ABSTRACT

Background/Objectives: Because no validated tool exists to assess nutrition knowledge regarding weight management we developed and tested the Weight Management Nutrition Knowledge Questionnaire (WMNKQ).

Subjects/Methods: The questionnaire assesses nutrition knowledge in these categories: energy density of food, portion size/serving size, alcohol and sugar sweetened beverages, how food variety affects food intake, and reliable nutrition information sources. Sixty questions were reviewed by 6 experts for face validity and quantitative analysis was used to assess item difficulty, item discrimination, internal consistency, inter-item-correlation, test-retest reliability, construct validity, criterion validity, and convergent validity.

Results: The final WMNKQ contained 43 items. Experts removed 3 of the original 60 questions and modified 41. Eighteen items did not meet criteria for item difficulty, item discrimination, and/or inter-item correlation; 4 were retained. The WMNKQ met criteria for internal consistency (Cronbach's alpha = 0.88), reliability (test-retest correlation ρ= 0.90, P <0.0001), construct validity (known groups comparison) - dietitians scored 16% better (p<0.0001) than information technology workers, and criterion validity (pre- to post-intervention improvement in knowledge scores = 11.2% (95% CI 9.8-12.5, p<0.0001)). Participants younger than age 55 scored significantly better than those over age 55 (convergent validity).

Conclusions: The WMNKQ measures how well nutrition principles of weight management are understood.

INTRODUCTION

The high prevalence[1] and associated medical costs of obesity in the United States provide an incentive to optimize obesity treatment, most often based upon comprehensive lifestyle interventions[2]. Factors contributing to fat gain include excess energy intake and low physical activity[3]. Some properties of food and food consumption patterns clearly contribute to excess energy intake. These include consumption of high energy dense foods[4, 5], large portion sizes[6], a greater variety of foods[7, 8] high in palatability[9], and sugar sweetened beverages[10]. Successful comprehensive lifestyle weight management programs help clients learn these nutrition concepts, teach cognitive behavior principles and support increased physical activity [2]. Most programs rely on the amount and duration of weight loss as the primary basis for evaluating success of all three components. There have been no systematic attempts to determine whether the nutritional knowledge components of these programs have been sufficiently well understood by the clients. When assessed, lifestyle programs used a general nutrition knowledge tool to measure knowledge[11].

Lack of success in losing weight may reflect inadequate teaching of important nutrition principles, failure to implement behavior change skills or both. We hypothesized that teaching nutrition principles would be more useful than asking clients to memorize a series of facts, because those who understand major concepts can apply them to novel situations not covered by a series of examples. A questionnaire that addresses knowledge related to the key dietary principles of successful weight management will allow programs to identify whether the nutrition education component has successfully transmitted fundamental concepts

Understanding nutrition principles does not necessarily guarantee behavioral changes that result in successful long term weight loss. However, the knowledge, attitude, and behavior[12, 13] model of health education implies that, although attitude is an important factor, it must be in conjunction with a gain in knowledge to result in successful behavior change. With the goal of evaluating the nutrition education component of our lifestyle intervention for obesity[14] we conducted a thorough literature review that involved a PubMed search using the key words "nutrition" or "nutritional" and "knowledge" and "questionnaire" or "survey" in the title. We found no validated instruments that tested dietary principles of weight management; instead, all published validated instruments tested general nutrition knowledge.

To address this gap, we developed a questionnaire that measures nutrition knowledge as it relates to weight management.

METHODS

The questionnaire will be referred to as the Weight Management Nutrition Knowledge Questionnaire (WMNKQ). We included questions regarding both the types of information that people should understand and potential sources of information to avoid. We did this because many of our patients rely on media that promotes products with no proven weight loss benefit [15]. As part of WMNKQ, we included two questions regarding sources of reliable nutrition information in order to allow future evaluations of whether knowledge of this topic can predict long-term weight management success. The aim of this report is to describe the development and validation steps for the WMNKQ. All protocols used to test the WMNKQ were reviewed and approved by the Mayo Clinic Institutional Review Board (IRB).

A pool of approximately 200 questions was developed by gathering items from published nutrition questionnaires and writing new items. The questions were designed so that as a whole they would assess the understanding of concepts, as opposed to a series of nutrition facts. We focused on areas of nutrition knowledge that are most specific to weight management - energy density of food, how portion size or serving size affects food intake, alcohol-containing and sugar sweetened beverages, the influence of the variety of available foods on food intake; we also included questions on reliable nutrition information sources.

Questions were gathered from different sources including the *Parmenter and J Wardle Questionnaire*[16], *NHLBI*[17], *CDC*[18], *Mayo Clinic Patient Education Center, and USDA*[19]. Permission to use one item modified from the Parmenter and J Wardle questionnaire[16], was granted by Springer Nature. We solicited questions and critiques from a registered dietitian and five scientists outside Mayo Clinic with recognized expertise in this field. The WMNKQ was designed for a 9th grade reading using the Flesch–Kincaid readability tests[20] level to ensure that the questions were clear, not confusing, non-debatable, and worded simply. We included questions in the five subtopic areas of nutrition knowledge mentioned above. By eliminating questions with similar content and those that were too complex or arcane, we reduced the item pool to 60 questions for further assessment.

Face validity:

Face validity refers to how relevant the items appear to be to the respondents[16]. These 60 questions were sent to six experts who were PhD or MD scientists working in the field of nutrition and registered dietitians for assessment of face validity. Experts were asked whether the topics covered were comprehensive within the domain of weight management specific nutrition knowledge and if the questions were unequivocal. They provided feedback for modifications, elimination and/or additions of questions. The draft after following these recommendations consisted of 57 items.

Quantitative assessment:

Two-hundred eighty-six adults residing in Olmsted County, MN (n=187) and Duval County, FL (n=99) completed the original 57 item questionnaire in person. Of the Olmsted County participants, 136 were recruited through Mayo Clinic campus advertisements and 51 were recruited from a church in Rochester, Minnesota. The 99 participants from Duval County were recruited at a health education event on Edward Waters College Campus. All participants were ≥18 years old and able to read/speak proficient English. All demographic data was self-reported, including BMI.

Validity Testing:

Construct validity is a psychometric test that determines the extent that an instrument is measuring what it is intended to measure[16]. Construct validity was assessed by using the 'known-groups method[21]' by administering the WMNKQ to 18 registered dietitians and 25 information technology (IT) specialists. Participants were recruited through flyer ads and website ads. These two groups have similar amounts of post-secondary education and we hypothesized they would differ in nutrition knowledge because of the nature of their careers. Independent sample t-tests were used to assess the difference in scores between groups, both for the overall questionnaire and for each section. Analysis of covariance was performed to control for demographic differences between the dietitians and IT specialists. Test-retest reliability was assessed by giving the questionnaire to the dietitians and IT specialists on two separate occasions two weeks apart. We then assessed the correlation between the scores obtained on the two occasions the questionnaire was administered.

In psychometric analysis of questionnaires, criterion validity testing is done to assess whether items in an instrument correlate with an expected outcome[22]. We hypothesized that an intervention designed to increase weight management nutrition knowledge would result in an increase in score on our questionnaire; this is a well-recognized approach to test for "criterion validity". Criterion validity was assessed by providing a nutrition knowledge intervention consisting of three, one-hour classes, to 119 participants of the Olmstead county cohort as part of the qualitative assessment component of this study. The materials used for the classes were developed and adapted from material used in the Look AHEAD trial[23]. Some content was created from materials developed by registered dietitians, a physician trained in nutrition and a clinical and translation science PhD doctoral student. The sessions were provided over a 1-2 week period to twelve groups of participants with approximately 10 participants per group. The sessions were designed to address the general concepts we identified as important for weight management without giving examples that are present in the questionnaire. The didactic content was delivered with PowerPoint presentations, hands on learning activities with food models, and 15 min for discussion, questions and answers. The WMNKQ was administered pre- and post-intervention. A $45 gift card incentive was given for attending all three sessions and completing both pre- and post-intervention questionnaires. Three different interventionists (two experienced weight management registered dietitian and a PhD student) taught the classes using identical materials; each interventionist taught four groups. The improvement in scores was compared for all participants and between the participants taught by the different interventionists to determine whether there was greater or lesser knowledge gain as a function of the interventionist to whom the participants were assigned. Changes in the results before and after the nutrition knowledge intervention class were compared to assess criterion validity of the questionnaire and for each section.

Convergent validity assesses whether expected associations exist between instrument responses and demographic variables that should differ between groups. If we observed the predicted correlations between age, education, and nutrition knowledge as assessed by our questionnaire we would take this "convergent validity" as additional evidence for the usefulness of WMNKQ. Convergent validity was assessed using data from 126 participants from Duval County and Olmsted County. We hypothesized that nutrition knowledge score would be greater in more educated participants[24] and in younger than to older participants[25]. Correlations between scores and demographic variables were examined. The association between nutrition knowledge scores with both age groups and education was assessed using analysis of covariance (ANCOVA).

Scoring System:

For validation purposes, the total score was expressed as a percentage correct. We also examined a weighted score system that may be more useful in guiding the nutrition teaching and evaluation of comprehensive lifestyle intervention programs. For this system the energy density questions are weighted as 40%, the portion size questions are weighed at 40% and the beverage section is weighted 20%. The questions on the topics of how food variety affects food intake and reliable nutrition information sources are scored separately

Statistical Analysis Methods

All analyses were performed utilizing two sided tests with the significance level alpha of set *a priori* at 0.05. We report the relevant P values and 95% confidence intervals. Binary analysis is given as proportions, and means are accompanied by standard deviations. Statistical power analyses were performed to determine the appropriate number of volunteers to recruit as part of the IRB approval process and prior to beginning each of these studies.

For item difficulty, Kline et al. suggested that items answered correctly by less than 20% or more than 80% are of limited value and should be discarded[26]. However, Parmenter et al. suggested a range of >30% and <90% for their nutrition knowledge questionnaire because they determined that their population had a higher than average nutrition knowledge[16]. We adopted the range of > 90% or < 30% correct answers because the Olmstead county population has higher than expected health literacy[27], which may confer higher nutrition knowledge. For Item discrimination, Kline, Streiner, and Norman[26, 28, 29] suggest that an items with an item-total score correlation of less than 0.2 can be discarded; we utilized this as our screening value. For inter-item correlation, we calculated the agreement in scores between every two items in the questionnaire. Questions with an r > 0.9 were flagged for being potentially redundant[26]. For internal consistency reliability, Klein suggested that the minimum requirement is ≥ 0.7[26, 30]. We calculated Cronbach's alpha for the questionnaire overall and for each section.

For construct validity testing, we used an independent t-test to compare overall mean between dietitians and IT and used an analysis of co-variance to correct for demographic differences. For test-retest reliability we used the Spearman's correlation to examine similarities in results from questionnaires filled out in a two week interval with no intervention; Kline[26] suggest a minimum requirement of ρ of 0.7 for test-retest reliability. For criterion validity, we utilized a paired t- test to examine changes in score from before to after the nutrition education intervention.

RESULTS

<u>Face Validity</u>

Of the original 200 items, 60 were selected based on face validity. Feedback was incorporated into the questionnaire and the initial draft consisted of 57 items. Three questions were eliminated because the items were considered too ambiguous or arcane.

Quantitative Analysis

Demographics for the participants from medical center and from Duval County are provided in Table 1. Eighteen items were flagged for possible exclusion based upon the criteria described in the Methods. Of those eighteen items, four were retained because they tested important concepts and were considered necessary in our questionnaire (see below).

Item difficulty:

Six items were deemed unhelpful in assessing weight management nutrition knowledge because they were answered correctly by greater than 90% of participants; all 6 were excluded.

Five items were answered correctly by less than 30% of participants; these could either be poorly worded (ambiguous) or were dealing with topics that are less common knowledge. Of these 5 items, 4 were excluded and 1 (number 34) was retained. Item 34 tested knowledge regarding the energy content of different alcoholic beverages. This item displayed the greatest single question improvement (56%) in score following the nutrition education intervention (see below), indicating that the low score reflected a lack of knowledge rather than difficult wording of the question. A total of 9 items were excluded on the basis of item difficulty.

Item discrimination:

Eight items had an item to total score correlation of less than 0.2. Three items were excluded and four (numbers 2, 6, 28 and 34) were retained. Item 2 tested knowledge of how adding low energy density food to a high energy density food can decrease the overall calories per serving, a concept that we deemed necessary to test. In addition, the improvement in score for this question was 29% following the intervention. Item 6 tested the knowledge of the "buffet effect," a concept that examines how the variety of foods available at a meal affects food intake. The improvement in score for this question was 27% following the nutrition education intervention. Item 28 likewise tested the concept that a larger number of food options at a meal increases the likelihood of consuming excess calories. The improvement in score of this question in response to the educational intervention was 40%. Item 34 was retained as described above.

Item to item correlation:

Two items had a score correlation of greater than 0.9 and were already excluded for not meeting item difficulty criteria.

Internal consistency:

Overall Cronbach's alpha for the remaining 43 items was 0.88. Cronbach's alpha for each category of questions is provided in Table 2.

Construct validity (known-groups comparison):

Eighteen dietitians and 25 IT workers completed the questionnaire; their demographics are provided in Table 3. The dietitians were mainly women and IT workers were mainly men. The dietitians scored an average of 92% (95% CI 90-95 %) and the average score for IT workers was 76% (95% CI 72 - 81%), for an overall difference of 16% (p<0.0001), which remained significant after adjusting for sex and income (Table 4). The dietitians did not score significantly better in the topic of how food variety affects food intake, however, there were only two questions on this topic.

Test-retest reliability:

The registered dietitians and IT workers were administered the questionnaire 14 +/-2 days apart. Spearman correlation for total score was ρ= 0.90, p<0.0001, indicating acceptable test-retest reliability (Table 5).

Criterion Validity

Of the original 286 participants, 136 enrolled in the nutrition knowledge intervention classes. Of these, 119 attended all 3 classes and completed the post-intervention questionnaire. For these participants the 57-item questionnaire was administered, but criterion validity was calculated using only the 43 final items. The improvement in overall scores was 11.2% (95% CI 9.8-12.5, p<0.0001, Table 6), indicating the questionnaire met the standards for criterion validity. Table 6 provides the differences in scores by topic. The improvement in scores was not different between the three interventionists (P = 0.35).

Two of the interventionists had no access to the survey for at least 6 months before they began teaching the classes. The third interventionist (DM) was responsible for providing the paper surveys to the participants and thus had access to the survey. Evidence that this does not invalidate the criterion validity results includes the lack of between-group differences and that the improvement in scores for those 79 participants taught by the first two interventionists was 11.6% (95% confidence interval 8.6% - 14.6%, P < 0.0001.

Based on the results of internal consistency, it was more reasonable to group specific sets of questions (Table 6). A weighted scoring algorithm was developed to use in future lifestyle intervention programs. Trustworthy nutrition information source and variety of food affects energy intake sections were not included in the weighted scoring algorithm to derive a total score because of their low internal consistency. The four questions included in these two sections remain in the questionnaire as standalone questions.

Convergent Validity

Consistent with our hypothesis, participants with undergraduate and graduate degrees scored significantly better on this questionnaire than those with a high school diploma or less (Table 7). Nutrition knowledge scores were also higher among the younger (age <35) and middle age (35-54) participants compared to the older participants (age ≥55).

DISCUSSION

We developed and tested the WMNKQ, a 43 item questionnaire that measures nutrition knowledge as it relates to weight management. We subjected our questionnaire to tests for item difficulty, item discrimination and item-to-item correlation in order to remove unnecessary questions. WMNKQ was tested using published criteria for internal consistency, construct validity using the known-groups comparison approach, test-retest reliability, criterion validity, and we found evidence for convergent validity. The results indicate that the WMNKQ is a useful tool that can assess nutrition knowledge relevant to weight management in order to determine how well-linked this knowledge is to long-term success.

Our results indicate that some types of energy intake concepts are not well-understood, but that deficits in these knowledge areas are readily correctable. Our participants scored < 50% correct in the categories of alcohol intake/sugar sweetened beverages and how variety of food affects energy intake. However, after attending classes to improve nutrition knowledge as it relates to weight management, scores on both sections improved significantly (table 6). The potential quantitative effects of these concepts are not trivial. Sixty-nine percent of US adults consume at least 255 Kcal/day from alcohol[31] and 49% consume at least one sugar sweetened beverage/day (average 145 Kcal/day)[32], which may contribute to excess energy intake and obesity[33, 34]. With respect to the potential effects of greater food variety, previous studies have shown that volunteers offered three food choices versus one consume ~20% more food[8]. Furthermore, consumption of a greater variety of energy dense foods is associated with overweight[35]. Thus, greater food variety is a quantitatively important contributor to excess energy intake. The WMNKQ should allow investigators to assess whether a better understanding of these two concepts is associated with greater success in weight management.

The category of energy density (19 questions)[36] was overemphasized in our questionnaire because of its quantitative importance in controlled studies[37]. A direct association between dietary energy density and weight gain has been shown[36]. We developed questions using food labels with calorie content and portion size to assess whether people can evaluate energy density information, including how fiber-rich foods relate to energy density. The second largest category in terms of questions (15 questions) was related to portion size, where we tested the understanding of serving size and standard portions, knowledge that is essential for achieving weight loss[38]. The ability to understand food labels[39, 40] was incorporated into several categories to determine whether knowledge deficits are related to food label understanding vs. the topic itself. We included 2 questions on "reliable nutrition information sources" because, although there is widespread availability of digital nutrition information, this information is often inaccurate[15]. We addressed this issue in our comprehensive lifestyle weight management program in response to participant feedback and chose to include questions that briefly assess knowledge of this topic. We hope to eventually understand whether a better understanding of what sources of nutrition information has predictive value for successful weight management. The topic(s) of alcohol/sugar sweetened beverages and how food variety affects energy intake[7, 41] were also less amenable to non-repetitive examples and we also included limited numbers of questions on these topics. This makes it difficult to perform all of the statistical analyses for the categories with fewer questions, however. That said, the analyses of the questionnaire overall support our contention that it can provide a useful tool to test for nutrition knowledge specific to weight management. Although, other nutrition knowledge questionnaires contain questions/sections related to weight management[15, 24, 42-45], our questionnaire is unique because it includes the above described five categories as they pertain to weight management.

Most nutrition knowledge questionnaires[16, 25, 42-45] examine general nutrition knowledge and undergo a series of validation tests[16, 25, 44, 45]. All 4 general nutrition knowledge questionnaires[16, 25, 42-45] underwent tests for construct validity, test-retest reliability and internal consistency. Item difficulty analysis was performed in the GNKQ, Jones, and the Feren questionnaires, but not the GNKQ-R. Item discrimination analysis was performed in the GNKQ, GNKQ-R, and the Jones questionnaires, but not in the Feren questionnaire. The GNKQ-R included tests for criterion validity and convergent validity. None of the questionnaires performed item to item correlation analysis. The WMNKQ underwent analysis and appropriate modifications when tested for item difficulty, item discrimination, item-to-item correlation and internal consistency. It met validity criteria for test-retest reliability, construct validity, criterion validity, and convergent validity. Thus, our evaluation of the WMNKQ was more stringent than the available general nutrition knowledge questionnaires.

As was done with other questionnaires[16, 25, 42-45], we retained some questions that did not meet the usual statistical criteria for difficulty or item discrimination. The retained questions had marked improvements in scores after a standardized weight management nutrition education intervention, suggesting that these knowledge domains are distinct and that deficits are correctable. The overall average improvement in score was 11%, whereas the 4 items we retained that did not meet usual criteria for inclusion demonstrated a much greater improvement in scores. If these items were worded in a difficult or ambiguous way, a nutrition knowledge intervention would likely not result in an improvement in score for these items. We propose that retaining knowledge-related items that don't meet the usual criteria for difficulty or item discrimination is acceptable if there is evidence from criteria validity assessment that the questions address areas of uncommon knowledge.

Improvement in scores following a nutritional knowledge intervention is important for questionnaire validation. We used several tactics to ensure that we were not teaching to the questionnaire. The presentations were developed around the topics, not the specific questions. Only one of the three interventionists was involved in question development and the interventionists were not allowed to have the questionnaire available around the time of the classes. Had an interventionist's specific knowledge of the questionnaire been an important factor in score improvement, the participants in that individual's classes should have outperformed the other two interventionists. Instead we found that the improvement in scores achieved by the participants was consistent between all three interventionists.

The test-retest reliability of the WMNKQ was highly statistically significant, with most sections demonstrating a Spearman correlation of $\rho= 0.7$ or greater (Table 5). The exception was for the section on how a variety of foods affects food intake, which only contained 2 questions. Gaining a high level of test-retest reliability with only 2 questions would require that over 43 persons would have to give the exact same answers for both questions. Therefore, it is very difficult to achieve a correlation of ≥ 0.70 with only two questions. The rational for including only two questions for this category is discussed above. The WMNKQ has acceptable test-retest reliability, as demonstrated by the test-retest correlation for the overall score of 0.90.

One limitation of the study is that the sample size power calculations were to test for statistical significance of the questionnaire as a whole and not for each subsection. Only 45 dietitians and information technologists participated in the test-retest and known group comparison validation tests, which limited the statistical power when analyzing *subsections* of the questionnaire. However, we were still able to demonstrate that the questionnaire is a robust tool. Another limitation of this study was that the Olmsted County participants were mostly white and for the most part more educated than volunteers from Duval County, which can introduce bias. However, upon convergent validity analysis nutrition knowledge was related to education level not race. Finally, the questionnaire is that it is designed for the adult population and was not tested in the pediatric or adolescent population. However, most participants in lifestyle intervention programs are older than 18.

The WMNKQ has multiple potential applications. It could be used to assess the effectiveness of nutrition knowledge interventions as part of interventional lifestyle programs. The WMNKQ may be useful to understand whether nutrition knowledge in the areas included in the questionnaire predicts long-term weight loss success. We acknowledge that gain in nutrition knowledge does not necessarily predict weight loss [46] because of the importance of the behavior change component necessary to translate the knowledge into action. The WMNKQ can potentially be used as a tool to help guide the allocation of public nutrition education efforts to different demographic areas. The scoring in sections of the questionnaires can pinpoint specific knowledge deficits to guide funds. We also plan to employ the questionnaire as part of patient intake prior to nutrition consultations to focus health education efforts towards closing specific knowledge gaps. In conclusion, we propose that the WMNKQ helps quantify the understanding of basic concepts in the areas of nutrition knowledge with respect to weight management and will provide a useful tool to test whether that knowledge relates to improved outcomes.

ACKNOWLEDGMENTS

We appreciate the help of Pam Reich for study coordination and the cooperation of our volunteers.

COMPETING INTERESTS

The authors declared no conflict of interest.

REFERENCES

1.   Ogden CL, Carroll MD, Kit BK, Flegal KM. Prevalence of obesity in the United States, 2009-2010. *NCHS Data Brief* 2012; **(82)**: 1-8.
2.   Jensen MD, Ryan DH, Apovian CM, Ard JD, Comuzzi AG, Donato KA, et al. 2013 AHA/ACC/TOS guideline for the management of overweight and obesity in adults: a report of the American College of Cardiology/American Heart Association Task Force on Practice Guidelines and The Obesity Society. *Circulation* 2014; **129(25 Suppl 2)**: S102-S38.
3.   Church TS, Thomas DM, Tudor-Locke C, Katzmarzyk PT, Earnest CP, Rodarte RQ, et al. Trends over 5 decades in U.S. occupation-related physical activity and their associations with obesity. *PLoS One* 2011; **6(5)**: e19657.
4.   Rolls BJ. The relationship between dietary energy density and energy intake. *Physiol Behav* 2009; **97(5)**: 609-15.
5.   Rouhani MH, Haghighatdoost F, Surkan PJ, Azadbakht L. Associations between dietary energy density and obesity: A systematic review and meta-analysis of observational studies. *Nutrition* 2016; **32(10)**: 1037-47.
6.   Ledikwe JH, Ello-Martin JA, Rolls BJ. Portion Sizes and the Obesity Epidemic. *J Nutr* 2005; **135(4)**: 905-9.
7.   Rolls BJ, Van Duijvenvoorde PM, Rowe EA. Variety in the diet enhances intake in a meal and contributes to the development of obesity in the rat. *Physiol Behav* 1983; **31(1)**: 21-7.
8.   Rolls BJ, Rowe EA, Rolls ET, Kingston B, Megson A, Gunary R. Variety in a meal enhances food intake in man. *Physiol Behav* 1981; **26(2)**: 215-21.
9.   McCrickerd K, Forde CG. Sensory influences on food intake control: moving beyond palatability. *Obes Rev* 2016; **17(1)**: 18-29.
10.   Schulze MB, Manson JE, Ludwig DS, Colditz GA, Stampfer MJ, Willett WC, et al. Sugar-sweetened beverages, weight gain, and incidence of type 2 diabetes in young and middle-aged women. *JAMA* 2004; **292(8)**: 927-34.
11.   Barbosa LB, Vasconcelos SM, Correia LO, Ferreira RC. Nutrition knowledge assessment studies in adults: a systematic review. *Ciencia & saude coletiva* 2016; **21(2)**: 449-62.
12.   Ajzen I. The theory of planned behaviour: reactions and reflections. *Psychology & health* 2011; **26(9)**: 1113-27.
13.   Fishbein M, Ajzen I. *Belief, attitude, intention and behaviour: An introduction to theory and research*, 27 ed. Addison-Wesley Pub. Co.: Reading, MA, 1975.
14.   Mikhail DS, Jensen T, B,, Wade TW, Myers JF, Frank JM, Wieland M, et al. Methodology of a multispecialty outpatient Obesity Treatment Program. *Contemporary Clinical Trials Communications* 2018; **10**: 36-41.
15.   Tonsaker T, Bartlett G, Trpkov C. Health information on the Internet: gold mine or minefield? *Canadian Family Physician Medecin de famille Canadien* 2014; **60(5)**: 407-8.
16.   Parmenter K, Wardle J. Development of a general nutrition knowledge questionnaire for adults. *Eur J Clin Nutr* 1999; **53(4)**: 298-308.
17.   National Heart, Lung, and Blood Institute. *Choosing Foods for Your Family*. 2013, May 17 [Available from: https://www.nhlbi.nih.gov/health/educational/wecan/eat-right/choosing-foods.htm].
18.   Centers for Disease Control and Prevention. *Healthy Eating for a Healthy Weight*. 2016, September 8 [Available from: https://www.cdc.gov/healthyweight/healthy_eating/index.html].

19.   United States Department of Agriculture. *Choose MyPlate*. 2018 January 31 [Available from: https://www.choosemyplate.gov/].

20.   Flesch R. A new readability yardstick. *JAppl Psychol* 1948; **32(3)**: 221-33.

21.   Hofman CS, Lutomski JE, Boter H, Buurman BM, de Craen AJ, Donders R, et al. Examining the construct and known-group validity of a composite endpoint for The Older Persons and Informal Caregivers Survey Minimum Data Set (TOPICS-MDS); A large-scale data sharing initiative. *PLoS One* 2017; **12(3)**: e0173081.

22.   Cordier R, Milbourn B, Martin R, Buchanan A, Chung D, Speyer R. A systematic review evaluating the psychometric properties of measures of social inclusion. *PLoS One* 2017; **12(6)**: e0179109.

23.   Ryan DH, Espeland MA, Foster GD, Haffner SM, Hubbard VS, Johnson KC, et al. Look AHEAD (Action for Health in Diabetes): design and methods for a clinical trial of weight loss for the prevention of cardiovascular disease in type 2 diabetes. *Control Clin Trials* 2003; **24(5)**: 610-28.

24.   Furnee CA, Groot W, van den Brink HM. The health effects of education: a meta-analysis. *Eur J Public Health* 2008; **18(4)**: 417-21.

25.   Kliemann N, Wardle J, Johnson F, Croker H. Reliability and validity of a revised version of the General Nutrition Knowledge Questionnaire. *Eur J Clin Nutr* 2016; **70(10)**: 1174-80.

26.   Kline P. *The handbook of psychological testing*. Routledge: London ; New York, 1993. vi, 627

27.   Fabbri M, Yost K, Finney Rutten LJ, Manemann SM, Boyd CM, Jensen D, et al. Health Literacy and Outcomes in Patients With Heart Failure: A Prospective Community Study. *Mayo Clin Proc* 2018; **93(1)**: 9-15.

28.   Streiner DL, Norman GR. *Health measurement scales : a practical guide to their development and use*, 2nd ed. Oxford University Press: Oxford ; New York, 1995. viii, 231 p. p.

29.   Everitt B, Skrondal A. *The Cambridge dictionary of statistics*, 4th ed. Cambridge University Press: Cambridge, UK ; New York, 2010. ix, 468

30.   Cronbach LJ, Meehl PE. Construct validity in psychological tests. *Psychol Bull* 1955; **52(4)**: 281-302.

31.   Organization WH. Alcohol Consumption Levels and Patterns. 2014.

32.   Rosinger A, Herrick K, Gahche J, Park S. Sugar-sweetened Beverage Consumption Among U.S. Adults, 2011-2014. *NCHS data brief* 2017; **(270)**: 1-8.

33.   Sayon-Orea C, Martinez-Gonzalez MA, Bes-Rastrollo M. Alcohol consumption and body weight: a systematic review. *Nutr Rev* 2011; **69(8)**: 419-31.

34.   Bebb HT, Houser HB, Witschi JC, Littell AS, Fuller RK. Calorie and nutrient contribution of alcoholic beverages to the usual diets of 155 adults. *Am J Clin Nutr* 1971; **24(9)**: 1042-52.

35.   Rolls BJ. The role of portion size, energy density, and variety in obesity and weight management. In: Wadden TA, Bray GA, editors. *Handbook of Obesity Treatment*. Second ed. New York, NY: The Guilford Press; 2018. p. 93-104.

36.   Ledikwe JH, Blanck HM, Kettel Khan L, Serdula MK, Seymour JD, Tohill BC, et al. Dietary energy density is associated with energy intake and weight status in US adults. *Am J Clin Nutr* 2006; **83(6)**: 1362-8.

37.   Flood JE, Rolls BJ. Soup preloads in a variety of forms reduce meal energy intake. *Appetite* 2007; **49(3)**: 626-34.

38.   Rolls BJ. What is the role of portion control in weight management? *Int J Obes (Lond)* 2014; **38 Suppl 1**: S1-8.

39.   Ollberding NJ, Wolf RL, Contento I. Food label use and its relation to dietary intake among US adults. *J Am Diet Assoc* 2010; **110(8)**: 1233-7.

40.	Satia JA, Galanko JA, Neuhouser ML. Food nutrition label use is associated with demographic, behavioral, and psychosocial factors and dietary intake among African Americans in North Carolina. *J Am Diet Assoc* 2005; **105(3)**: 392-402; discussion -3.
41.	Norton GN, Anderson AS, Hetherington MM. Volume and variety: relative effects on food intake. *Physiol Behav* 2006; **87(4)**: 714-22.
42.	Pellegrini N, Salvatore S, Valtuena S, Bedogni G, Porrini M, Pala V, et al. Development and validation of a food frequency questionnaire for the assessment of dietary total antioxidant capacity. *J Nutr* 2007; **137(1)**: 93-8.
43.	Obayashi S, Bianchi LJ, Song WO. Reliability and validity of nutrition knowledge, social-psychological factors, and food label use scales from the 1995 Diet and Health Knowledge Survey. *J Nutr Educ Behav* 2003; **35(2)**: 83-91.
44.	Jones AM, Lamp C, Neelon M, Nicholson Y, Schneider C, Wooten Swanson P, et al. Reliability and validity of nutrition knowledge questionnaire for adults. *J Nutr Educ Behav* 2015; **47(1)**: 69-74.
45.	Feren A, Torheim LE, Lillegaard IT. Development of a nutrition knowledge questionnaire for obese adults. *Food Nutr Res* 2011; **55**.
46.	Worsley A. Nutrition knowledge and food consumption: can nutrition knowledge change food behaviour? *Asia Pac J Clin Nutr* 2002; **11 Suppl 3**: S579-85.

Table 1: Socio-demographic characteristics of Olmsted County and Duval County volunteers

	Olmsted County Volunteers (N=187)	Duval County Volunteers (N=99)
Age (years)		
Younger: <35	50	30
Middle age: 35-54	52	30
Older: >=55	22	39
Sex		
Male	30	20
Female	96	78
Race/Ethnicity		
White	101	3
Black, African American, or African descent	2	86
Hispanic/Latino(a)/ or Spanish origin	8	3
American Indian or Alaska Native	0	3
Asian	13	0
Hawaiian or other Pacific Islander	1	1
Multiple races	0	3
Marital Status		
Single	44	51
Married	74	22
Widowed/Divorced/Separated	7	26
Education		
High School or less	8	40

Undergraduate	85	27
Graduate	31	32
BMI		
Normal	38	30
Overweight	40	21
Obese	40	46

Some participants were not asked to provide demographic information. These characteristics are self-reported.

BMI - Body Mass Index

Table 2: Internal consistency the overall questionnaire and individual sections

	Cronbach's Alpha
Overall Cronbach's Alpha (43 items)	0.88
Energy Density (19 items)	0.78
Portion Size (15 items)	0.74
Variety of Food Affects Food Intake (2 items)	0.18
Reliable Nutrition Information Source (2 items)	0.23
Alcohol Intake and Sugar Sweetened Beverages (5 items)	0.44

Table 3: Socio-demographic characteristics of dietitians and information technologists

	Dieticians (N=18)	IT* (N=25)	Total (N=43)	p value
Age				0.0679
25-34 years old	6 (33%)	1 (4%)	7 (16%)	
35-44 years old	4 (22%)	12 (48%)	16 (37%)	
45-54 years old	3 (17%)	7 (28%)	10 (23%)	
55-64 years old	4 (22%)	3 (12%)	7 (16%)	
65-74 years old	1 (6%)	2 (8%)	3 (7%)	
Sex				0.0003
Male	1 (6%)	15 (60%)	16 (37%)	
Female	17 (94%)	10 (40%)	27 (63%)	
Race				0.2044
White	18 (100%)	21 (84%)	39 (91%)	
Black, African American, or African descent	0 (0%)	1 (4%)	1 (2%)	
Asian	0 (0%)	3 (12%)	3 (7%)	
Marital Status				0.8834
Single	2 (11%)	4 (16%)	6 (14%)	
Married	15 (83%)	20 (80%)	35 (81%)	
Divorced	1 (6%)	1 (4%)	2 (5%)	
Education				0.6972
Undergraduate	9 (50%)	14 (56%)	23 (53%)	
Graduate	9 (50%)	11 (44%)	20 (47%)	
Income				0.4337
$40,000-$49,999	1 (6%)	0 (0%)	1 (2%)	
$50,000-$74,999	3 (17%)	2 (8%)	5 (12%)	
$75,000-$99,999	2 (11%)	4 (16%)	6 (14%)	
$100,000-$150,000	7 (39%)	14 (56%)	21 (49%)	
Over $150,000	2 (11%)	4 (16%)	6 (14%)	
Would rather not say	3 (17%)	1 (4%)	4 (9%)	
BMI Group**				0.0080
Missing	0	1	1	
Underweight	1 (6%)	0 (0%)	1 (2%)	
Normal	15 (83%)	9 (38%)	24 (57%)	
Overweight	1 (6%)	8 (33%)	9 (21%)	
Obese	1 (6%)	7 (29%)	8 (19%)	

There was no statistically significant difference in demographic variables except for BMI

and sex. ANCOVA was used to adjusting for sex and income.

IT = Information Technologist; BMI = Body Mass Index

Table 4: Differences in nutrition knowledge scores between dietitians and information technologists

	Dietitians (N=18)	IT (N=25)	p value
Total Score			<0.0001
Mean (SD)	39.7 (2.5)	32.8 (5.1)	
% Correct (43 Items)	92.3%	76.3%	
Energy Density			0.0001
Mean (SD)	18.4 (1.0)	14.9 (3.4)	
% Correct (19 Items)	96.8%	78.4%	
Portion Size			0.0004
Mean (SD)	13.3 (1.1)	11.5 (1.8)	
% Correct (15 Items)	88.7%	76.7%	
Variety of food affects food intake			0.8850
Mean (SD)	1.1 (0.8)	1.1 (0.6)	
% Correct (2 Items)	55.0	55.0	
Reliable nutrition information source			0.0034
Mean (SD)	2.0 (0.0)	1.6 (0.5)	
% Correct (2 Items)	100%	80.0%	
Alcohol and Sugar Sweetened Beverages			0.0001
Mean (SD)	4.8 (0.4)	3.7 (1.0)	
% Correct (5 Items)	98.0%	74.0%	

Construct validity was evaluated using the "known-groups method". Percentage difference in scores for Dietitians and IT from the first time they completed the questionnaire was calculated for the overall questionnaire and for each section. The mean and percentage correct was based on the number of questions per section. Independent t-test was used to assess the differences between groups.

Table 5: Test-retest reliability

Categories	Spearman Correlation (ρ)	p-value
Total Score	0.90	<.0001
Energy Density	0.94	<.0001
Portion Size	0.74	<.0001
Variety of Food Affects Food Intake	0.53	0.0002
Reliable Nutrition Information Source	0.70	<.0001
Alcohol Intake + Sugar Sweetened Beverages	0.67	<.0001

The time interval between the two times the questionnaire was administered was 2 weeks +/- 3 days. Test-retest reliability was assessed by giving the questionnaire to a total of 45 dietitians and IT specialists. Spearman Correlation for total score and for each section was calculated.

Table 6: Differences in knowledge scores pre- and post-intervention of Olmsted County Sample

	Pre Intervention Results (%)	Post Intervention Results (%)	P Value
Overall Score	75.4; 95% CI [73.4, 77.3]	86.6; 95% CI [85.2, 88.1]	<0.0001
Alcohol Intake and Sugar Sweetened Beverages	70.0; 95% CI [65.0, 75.2]	85.4; 95% CI [83.5, 87.3]	<0.0001
Energy Density	76.6; 95% CI [73.7, 79.4]	85.7; 95% CI [81.1, 90.2]	<0.0001
Portion Size	77.1; 95% CI [74.0, 80.3]	86.89; 95% CI [84.6, 89.2]	<0.0001
Reliable Nutrition Information	82.4; 95% CI [79.2, 85.6]	92.4; 95% CI [91.2, 93.7]	<0.0002
Variety of Food Affects Food Intake	57.1; 95% CI [54.8, 59.5]	91.2; 95% CI [90.4, 91.9]	<0.0001
Overall Weighted Score*	75.5%	86.1%	<0.0001

Three one hour nutrition knowledge weight management education intervention was administered to 119 participants of the Olmstead County. The questionnaire was administered pre- and post-nutrition class intervention. Paired t-test was used to assess mean difference in score pre and post nutrition knowledge intervention.

*For the overall weighted score, energy density was given a 40% weight, portion size given a 40% weight, and alcohol intake and sugar sweetened beverages was given a 20% of the overall questionnaire. Reliable nutrition Information and variety of food affects food intake were not included in the weighted score and were treated as stand alone questions.

Table 7: Convergent validity assessing the correlation between nutrition knowledge score and demographic variables

	Younger: <35 (N=80)	Middle Age: 35-54 (N=82)	Older: >=55 (N=60)	Total (N=222)	p value
Total Score					0.0023
N	80	82	60	222	
Mean (SD	29.7 (6.4)	28.2 (7.6)	24.9 (8.1)	27.8 (7.6)	
Median	30.5	30.0	25.0	29.0	

	Graduate (N=62)	High School or Lower (N=48)	Undergraduate (N=112)	Total (N=222)	p value
Total Score					<0.0001
N	62	48	112	222	
Mean (SD	28.4 (7.6)	20.8 (6.6)	30.4 (6.0)	27.8 (7.6)	
Median	29.0	20.0	32.0	29.0	

Mean scores for different education and age groups are presented. ANCOVA was used to evaluate differences in score among different age groups. Younger and middle age groups are associated with higher nutrition knowledge. Independent t-test was used to evaluate differences in scores between education levels. Higher education levels are associated with higher mean scores.

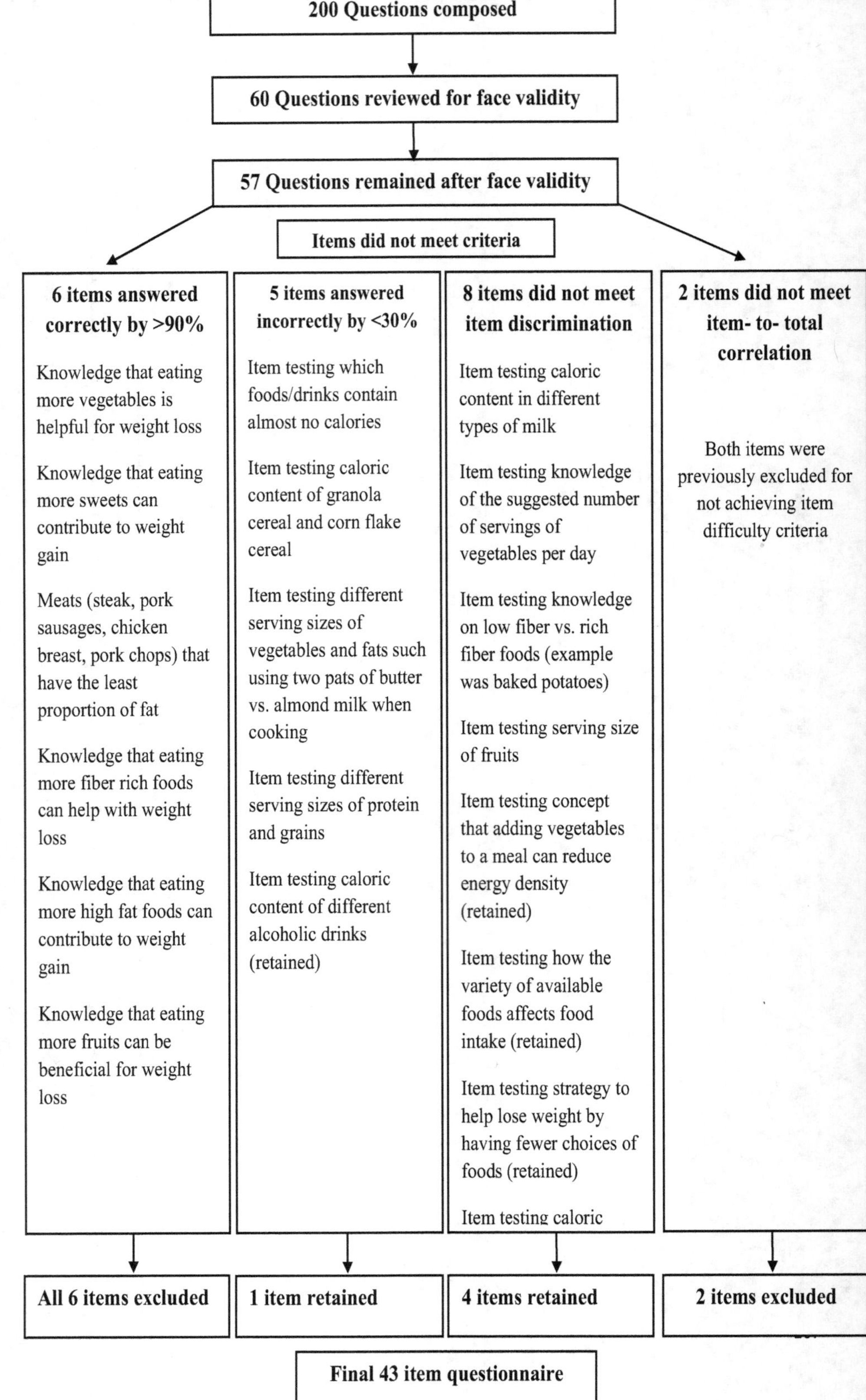

200 Questions composed

60 Questions reviewed for face validity

57 Questions remained after face validity

Items did not meet criteria

6 items answered correctly by >90%

Knowledge that eating more vegetables is helpful for weight loss

Knowledge that eating more sweets can contribute to weight gain

Meats (steak, pork sausages, chicken breast, pork chops) that have the least proportion of fat

Knowledge that eating more fiber rich foods can help with weight loss

Knowledge that eating more high fat foods can contribute to weight gain

Knowledge that eating more fruits can be beneficial for weight loss

5 items answered incorrectly by <30%

Item testing which foods/drinks contain almost no calories

Item testing caloric content of granola cereal and corn flake cereal

Item testing different serving sizes of vegetables and fats such using two pats of butter vs. almond milk when cooking

Item testing different serving sizes of protein and grains

Item testing caloric content of different alcoholic drinks (retained)

8 items did not meet item discrimination

Item testing caloric content in different types of milk

Item testing knowledge of the suggested number of servings of vegetables per day

Item testing knowledge on low fiber vs. rich fiber foods (example was baked potatoes)

Item testing serving size of fruits

Item testing concept that adding vegetables to a meal can reduce energy density (retained)

Item testing how the variety of available foods affects food intake (retained)

Item testing strategy to help lose weight by having fewer choices of foods (retained)

Item testing caloric

2 items did not meet item- to- total correlation

Both items were previously excluded for not achieving item difficulty criteria

All 6 items excluded

1 item retained

4 items retained

2 items excluded

Final 43 item questionnaire

Fig. 1 Outline of the validation steps followed in the development of the nutrition knowledge questionnaire. A total of 18 items did not fulfill criteria for item difficulty, item discrimination, and or inter-item correlation. Four of these items were retained. Although item 34 did not fulfill criteria for item difficulty and item discrimination, it was retained because it was only one of two items to address energy content of alcoholic beverages.

CHAPTER 5

DISCUSSION AND CONCLUSION

SUMMARY

Obesity is a global epidemic; approximately 160 million of the United States population is overweight or obese. Obesity is a health concern because it increases the risk for cardiovascular diseases and diabetes[1]. Lifestyle interventions provide an effective therapeutic treatment option for weight loss. Comprehensive lifestyle interventions are the cornerstone of obesity management and are prescribed as first-line treatment. Comprehensive lifestyle programs focus on cognitive behavioral interventions to achieve long-term positive changes in physical activity and nutrient intake. Long-term efficacy of lifestyle interventions is poor; insufficient weight loss has been documented and long-term sustainability is uncommon[2]. My overall goal was to develop and adapt methods that will systematically assess and improve the nutrition education component of a lifestyle intervention.

Aim 1:

To describe the methods of establishing a high intensity, year-long, comprehensive lifestyle treatment program for the medical management of obesity at Mayo Clinic, Rochester, MN.

Aim 2:

To report and evaluate the outcomes of the Obesity Treatment Research Program to provide a benchmark for subsequent program improvement interventions.

Aim 3:

To develop a novel weight management nutrition knowledge questionnaire (WMNKQ) that assesses nutrition knowledge as it relates to weight management. The survey will focus on the nutritional dimensions of five key areas: (1) portion size[3,4], (2) energy density of foods[5,6], (3) variety of food affect intake[7,8], (4) alcohol and sugar-sweetened beverages[9,10], (5) reliable nutrition information sources.

DISCUSSION

We herein investigated the best way to implement a comprehensive lifestyle intervention and outlined the most appropriate methods for data collection. In doing so, it described results from the obesity treatment research program. In chapter one, we describe the multi-specialty comprehensive lifestyle obesity program at Mayo Clinic in Rochester, Minnesota. This one-year high-intensity program focused included a nutritional intervention designed to reduce energy intake, a physical activity program and a cognitive behavioral approach to increase the likelihood of long-term adherence[11]. In chapter two, we investigated the weight loss outcomes for all the participants who enrolled in the program. We also used electronic medical records to collect follow-up data at one year and two years. The final chapter of this thesis, I discuss the development of a weight management questionnaire augmented by nutritional knowledge specific to participant needs.

One of the main findings of this study is that by getting informed consent to use the Mayo Clinic EMR we had the ability to collect one year weight measurements for 97% of OTRP participants and 83% at two years. Weight loss was modest in both completers and drop out; 38% of participants in a one year program lost at least 5% of their original body weight and 17`% lost at least 10%. After two years of program enrollment, 27% of participants lost at least 5% of their original body weight and approximately 6% of participants had at least a 10% reduction in weight. Although weight loss was modest, weight loss as little as 3-5% can result in clinically meaningful reductions in triglycerides, blood glucose, hemoglobin A1c (HbA1c), and the risk of developing type 2 diabetes[12].

Another major finding was that participants had low scores in two categories of nutritional knowledge: alcohol/sugar-sweetened beverages and how the variety of food affects food intake. Post-nutrition education intervention scores for both sections improved and were comparable to average scores on all other questions. The average improvement in scores for all questions in the WMNKQ was 11.2%. The items retained (4, 9, 27 and 37) demonstrated improved scores of 29%, 27%, 40%, and 56% respectively. These results suggest that knowledge deficits in alcohol intake and sugar-sweetened beverages and how the variety of food affects food intake are potentially widespread and easily correctable targets for comprehensive lifestyle interventions.

The results from comprehensive lifestyle interventions have been suboptimal. Development of methods to systematically evaluate and improve these interventions, therefore, remains a top clinical priority. We aim to advance the field through the design of a comprehensive lifestyle intervention plan taking into account obesity guidelines and recommendations, as well as through its thorough data collection element. Previous intervention plan attempts have failed to include these components.

We developed and validated the first instrument that tests nutrition knowledge specifically related to weight management. It is important for participants to understand food labels to be successful with weight management[13], and this is one of the main reasons we incorporated this into multiple sections of the questionnaire. All of these tested topics make the WMNKQ unique because the questions allow us to test the person's ability to use concepts to answer questions rather than memorize a series of facts. We also subjected the questionnaire to a robust validation process. The end result was a novel questionnaire with multiple clinical applications that can be both implemented in the field and used to create future iterations of nutritional knowledge assessments.

To date, almost all nutrition program assessments evaluate the combination of knowledge and behavior as outcome variables and, when the results are poor, assume the failure is in the behavior domain. Although this may be correct, it is possible that patients do change their behaviors but make equally poor nutrition choices because of insufficient conceptual understanding. The developed nutrition knowledge questionnaire herein was therefore developed using current literature, Mayo Survey Research Center expertise, and psychometric testing (face validity, construct validity, test-retest reliability, etc.). The intent behind this design was to create a questionnaire capable of determining to what extent gaps in knowledge contribute to less than desirable outcomes in regard to weight loss. Collecting data on participants knowledge gaps will serve to improve outcomes of comprehensive lifestyle treatment programs as a whole.

By comparing the before and after results of the survey following the educational intervention in our cohort, we gained unique insight into knowledge deficiencies that exist in the educational curriculum. By developing this questionnaire, we were able to measure nutrition knowledge among US adults across three different sites. By developing this questionnaire, we were able to develop a curriculum to fix knowledge gaps within different populations. This study is significant because there are no existing tools that measure nutrition knowledge specifically related to weight management.

Thesis as it pertains to clinical and translational science

The research in this thesis applies scientific principles of clinical translation science through a significant collaboration between clinical and scientific teams. Typically, lifestyle interventions involve administering a behavior health intervention, an exercise program, and a nutrition education program. However, this study's design enabled us to collect multiple data points throughout the one-year program, as well as an exhaustive list of questionnaires. In essence, the research plan was robust and was embedded within a clinical intervention to ultimately improve weight loss in overweight and obese participants.

This showcases the relationship between clinical teams and research teams for the ultimate benefit of the patient. The research plan was also developed as platform for other investigators to gather preliminary data for future bench to bedside research.

The nutrition knowledge questionnaire developed in this thesis highlights certain aspects of nutrition knowledge that are not widespread. This allowed the study team to move research knowledge or bedside conversations into the mainstream clinical forefront. Future application of this tool has significant clinical promise. For example, a clinician can utilize the WMNKQ as part of patient intake in the clinic setting, and use the results to guide time spent with their patients both in the clinic and potentially in lifestyle interventions. The questionnaire can give the clinician or dietitian information about the level of knowledge that patient has in areas such as understanding food labels or alcohol and sweetened beverage intake. The questionnaire would highlight these knowledge deficits, and contribute to effective bedside patient education. This is another example of how the work in this thesis incorporates clinical translational science principles.

Limitation of thesis

The original protocol of the OTRP was to enroll 500 participants over the course of five years, but due to lack of funding we were able to enroll only 156 participants. Despite this having an effect on the overall statistical power of the OTRP, we were still able to demonstrate statistically significant results with regards to weight loss following the intervention. A total of 8 groups were enrolled and a statistically significant weight loss outcome and decrease hip and waist circumference was reported in chapter two. However, we were not able to detect a statistically significant difference in neck circumference reduction (P=0.12). Most importantly, we learned how to organize and deliver an effective lifestyle intervention program, extract data using EMR data, and deliver online psychological surveys. These were all important goals achieved by establishing the OTRP. Another limitation of the study is not testing the questionnaire in the OTRP population. Clinical observations during the implementation of the OTRP led us to develop the WMNKQ; we were not able to implement the WMNKQ in the OTRP subjects because the OTRP study was finalized before the development of the WMNKQ was completed. However, we believe that this does not limit its use in future lifestyle interventions since the validations process highlights the questionnaires ability to test nutrition knowledge. The subjects in this project, although representative of the general public across the United States, do not represent the full spectrum of demographics. Olmsted County's population has higher than average health literacy and higher than average educational background when compared to the general public[14]. Duval County, an underserved population, was also unrepresentative of the general population of the United States. These two population extremes limit the generalizability of results.

Future directions

<u>The future direction of Aim 1 and 2</u>

Future directions could include consideration of investigating other avenues to evaluate and improve the ORTP. We have extensively discussed the nutrition knowledge component, evaluating, and improving throughout the dissertation, it is important to consider the other two arms of a comprehensive interventional lifestyle; physical activity and cognitive behavioral therapy.

There are different areas of physical activity assessments that are potentially worthwhile to investigate: first to potentially investigate the importance of increasing physical activity knowledge specific to weight management. There are many categories of physical activity concepts that are important to master for patients trying to manage or lose weight (1) importance of aerobic exercise and heart rate elevation in burning calories[15], (2) how to calculate calories burnt from specific physical activities, (3) expert recommendations on physical activity as its relationship to weight loss (4) reliable sources of physical activity information. Another area of assessment could involve developing reliable methods to assess the efficacy of exercise programs. It is important to measure subjects' adherence and compliance with the proposed exercise programs. A questionnaire to assess physical activity knowledge alone might not be sufficient; a novel method is needed to track physical activity progress and adherence.

Another future project is evaluating the cognitive behavioral health component of the ORTP; recent behavioral health research sheds light on the potential [16,17]. Multiple behavior models have been used to describe eating patterns[18,19]. Different methods to potentially modify excessive caloric consumption deserve additional research, and the design of an instrument to evaluate psychological eating behavior, addictive behaviors, and/or trends that are linked to excessive caloric consumption would be extremely valuable. Such a tool could be valuable to better identify and quantify pathological excessive caloric consumption behavior. Numerical tools also have the added benefit of being able to reveal changes in scores following an intervention. In summary, developing a tool to evaluate the efficacy of the behavioral health component of a lifestyle intervention can be very valuable.

<u>Future directions for the WMNKQ:</u>

There are multiple potential applications and future directions pertaining to this questionnaire. First, the questionnaire can be used in comprehensive lifestyle interventions to demonstrate pre-and post-intervention changes and to assess if post-intervention knowledge gaps persist. Moreover, in the future, the questionnaire can be used for lifestyle interventions in different populations, for example in adolescent, elderly, or even among other minority groups in the USA. Furthermore, the questionnaire can be translated into different languages (Spanish, French, German, etc.) and can be validated and used in the respective communities. This survey can also undergo further editing and translation to be suitable for use in third world countries such as sub-Saharan African countries; this might require substantial editing to suit the cultural, nutritional, and educational background of these populations. This editing, however, would entail further validation to ensure that the edited version still meets required biometric criteria.

REFERENCES

1.   Go, A.S., *et al.* Executive summary: heart disease and stroke statistics--2014 update: a report from the American Heart Association. *Circulation* **129**, 399-410 (2014).

2.   Jensen, M.D., *et al.* 2013 AHA/ACC/TOS guideline for the management of overweight and obesity in adults: a report of the American College of Cardiology/American Heart Association Task Force on Practice Guidelines and The Obesity Society. *Circulation* **129**, S102-138 (2014).

3.   Ledikwe, J.H., Ello-Martin, J.A. & Rolls, B.J. Portion Sizes and the Obesity Epidemic. *The Journal of Nutrition* **135**, 905-909 (2005).

4.   Livingstone, M.B.E. & Pourshahidi, L.K. Portion Size and Obesity. *Advances in Nutrition* **5**, 829-834 (2014).

5.   Duncan, K.H., Bacon, J.A. & Weinsier, R.L. The effects of high and low energy density diets on satiety, energy intake, and eating time of obese and nonobese subjects. *The American journal of clinical nutrition* **37**, 763-767 (1983).

6.   Rolls, B.J. The relationship between dietary energy density and energy intake. *Physiology & behavior* **97**, 609-615 (2009).

7.   Rolls, B.J., *et al.* Variety in a meal enhances food intake in man. *Physiology & behavior* **26**, 215-221 (1981).

8.   Rolls, B.J., Van Duijvenvoorde, P.M. & Rowe, E.A. Variety in the diet enhances intake in a meal and contributes to the development of obesity in the rat. *Physiology & behavior* **31**, 21-27 (1983).

9.   Welsh, J.A., Lundeen, E.A. & Stein, A.D. The sugar-sweetened beverage wars: public health and the role of the beverage industry. *Current opinion in endocrinology, diabetes, and obesity* **20**, 401-406 (2013).

10.   Worsley, A. Perceived reliability of sources of health information. *Health Education Research* **4**, 367-376 (1989).

11.   Mikhail, D.S., *et al.* Methodology of a multispecialty outpatient Obesity Treatment Research Program. *Contemporary clinical trials communications* **10**, 36-41 (2018).

12.   Donnelly, J.E., *et al.* American College of Sports Medicine Position Stand. Appropriate physical activity intervention strategies for weight loss and prevention of weight regain for adults. *Medicine and science in sports and exercise* **41**, 459-471 (2009).

13.   Rothman, R.L., *et al.* Patient understanding of food labels: the role of literacy and numeracy. *American journal of preventive medicine* **31**, 391-398 (2006).

14.   Fabbri, M., *et al.* Health Literacy and Outcomes in Patients With Heart Failure: A Prospective Community Study. *Mayo Clinic proceedings* **93**, 9-15 (2018).

15.   Swift, D.L., Houmard, J.A., Slentz, C.A. & Kraus, W.E. Effects of aerobic training with and without weight loss on insulin sensitivity and lipids. *PloS one* **13**, e0196637 (2018).

16.   Barry, D., Clarke, M. & Petry, N.M. Obesity and its relationship to addictions: is overeating a form of addictive behavior? *The American journal on addictions* **18**, 439-451 (2009).

17.   Ziauddeen, H., Farooqi, I.S. & Fletcher, P.C. Obesity and the brain: how convincing is the addiction model? *Nature reviews. Neuroscience* **13**, 279-286 (2012).

18.	Savage, J.S., Fisher, J.O. & Birch, L.L. Parental influence on eating behavior: conception to adolescence. *The Journal of law, medicine & ethics : a journal of the American Society of Law, Medicine & Ethics* **35**, 22-34 (2007).

19.	Doerksen, S.E. & McAuley, E. Social cognitive determinants of dietary behavior change in university employes. *Frontiers in public health* **2**, 23 (2014).

APPENDIX 1

Section A: Energy density of foods

1. To help reduce body fat, do you think heath experts recommend that people should eat more, the same, or less of these foods? (check one box per food)

	More	Same	Less
Vegetables (celery, carrots, green beans, etc.)			
Sweet foods (cookies, cakes, candy, etc.)			
Meats (steaks, chicken, fish, etc.)			
Foods high in starch (bread, potatoes, rice, etc.)			
Foods high in fat (ice cream, bacon, fried foods, etc.)			
Foods high in fiber (oat bran, black beans, squash, etc.)			
Fruits (apples, oranges, peaches etc.)			

2. Do you think these are high or low in fibers/ roughage? (check one box per food)

	High	Low
Raspberries		
Bananas		

Eggs		
Red meat		
Broccoli		
Green peas		
Lentils/beans		
Baked potatoes		
Fish		
Artichoke		

3. Which one of the following has the most calories for the same weight? (circle one)
   A. Table sugar
   B. Starchy foods (potato, bread)
   C. Foods with lots of fiber/ roughage
   D. Fat (butter, cooking oil)

4. Which would be the best choice for a low fat, high fiber light meal? (circle one)
   A. Grilled chicken
   B. Cheese on whole wheat toast
   C. Beans on whole wheat toast
   D. Quiche

5. Which of these meats has the least amount of fat? (circle one)
   A. grilled steak
   B. grilled pork sausages
   C. grilled turkey
   D. fried pork chop

6. According to the United States Department of Agriculture (USDA), what is the suggested amount of vegetables per day for a healthy diet? (circle one)
   A. ½ cup
   B. 1 ½ cups
   C. 2 ½ cups
   D. 5 cups

7. According to the United States Department of Agriculture (USDA), what is the suggested amount of fruits per day for a healthy diet? (circle one)
   A. 1 cup
   B. 2 cups
   C. 4 cups
   D. 6 cups

8. Which of these do not contain any Calories? (circle all that apply)
    A. Salt and pepper
    B. Fiber
    C. Skim milk
    D. Unsweetened tea
    E. Non- fat crackers

9. Which of the following foods has the most Calories? (circle one)
    A. 2 cups of spinach
    B. 1 tablespoon of olive oil
    C. 1 small cucumbers
    D. 1 small slice of whole wheat bread

10. If you are cooking ground beef, adding vegetables to the meal will: (circle one)
    A. Increase the amount of calories you are eating per 8 ounce serving
    B. Decrease the amount of calories you are eating per 8 ounce serving
    C. You are eating the same amount of calories per 8 ounce serving

11. What do you think the term "Calorie-dense foods" means? (circle one)
    A. Foods that have a lot of calories within smaller portions
    B. Foods that weigh more
    C. Foods that you have to eat a lot of to get enough calories

12. Eating fruits, legumes and vegetables can help you lose weight because? (circle one)
    A. They contain a lot of water
    B. They contain a lot of fiber
    C. Both A and B are correct
    D. They contain vitamins and antioxidants that help you lose weight

13. Which of the following has fewer calories? (circle one)
    A. 2 cups of vegetable beef stew
    B. 2 cups of vegetable beef soup
    C. 2 cups of vegetable beef lasagna
    D. They are all the same

14. Which of these strategies decreases the amount of calories you might eat for a meal? (circle all that applies)
    A. Choosing smaller portions of each food
    B. Using mustard on a sandwich instead of mayonnaise
    C. Substituting vegetables for pasta in a casserole
    D. Removing the skin from a chicken breast

15. If served 100 calories of each of these foods, which would give the largest portion?
    A. 1% fat cottage cheese
    B. Roasted chicken breast with the skin removed
    C. Tomato soup
    D. Blueberries

Section B: Sugar sweetened beverages

16. Which of these has the fewest Calories? (circle one)
    A. Cranberry apple cocktail
    B. Diet Cola
    C. Energy drink
    D. Dark chocolate mocha

17. Which of these coffee drinks is the lowest in calories?
    A. 12 fluid ounce latte with whole milk, syrup
    B. 12 fluid ounce latte with skim milk, sugar free syrup
    C. 12 fluid ounce latte with 2% milk, syrup
    D. 12 fluid ounce latte with almond milk, sugar free syrup

18. Which of these contains fewer calories per cup? (circle one)
    A. Fruit Juice
    B. A regular (non-diet) soda
    C. Skimmed milk

19. Which of the following has very few or no calories? (circle all that applies)
    A. Freshly brewed coffee with no sugar or milk
    B. Peach flavored herbal tea with no sugar added
    C. Freshly brewed tea with no sugar added
    D. Freshly squeezed cranberry juice with no sugar added
    E. Skimmed milk

20. If you are trying to lose weight, do you think it is helpful to drink a cup of fresh orange juice with each meal? (circle one)
A. True
B. False

Section C: How variety of foods affect food intake

21. Which of these is a good strategy to help to lose weight? (circle one)
    A. Having small number (<3) of foods to choose from per meal
    B. Having an average number (about5) of foods to choose from per meal
    C. Having a large number (>7) of foods to choose from per meal

22. You are on vacation and two different buffet style options are available for breakfast. **Buffet A** offers s a variety of fruits and vegetables. **Buffett B** offers a variety of fruits, vegetables, dairy products, and whole grain bakeries. If you want to lose weight, what should you do? (circle one)
    A. Pick Buffett A because it has less of a variety
    B. Pick Buffett B because it has more of a variety
    C. It doesn't matter which buffet because the amount of food consumed will probably be the same.

Section D: Portion size

23. According to the United Sates Department of Agriculture (USDA), a typical man will eat how many Calories per day to maintain his weight (circle one)
    A. 1,200- 1,600 Calories
    B. 1,800- 2,200 Calories
    C. 2,400- 2,800 Calories
    D. 3,000- 3,400 Calories

24. According to the United Sates Department of Agriculture (USDA), a typical woman will eat how many Calories per day to maintain her weight (circle one)
    A. 1,200- 1,600 Calories
    B. 1,800- 2,200 Calories
    C. 2,400- 2,800 Calories
    D. 3,000- 3,400 Calories

25. According to the United Sates Department of Agriculture (USDA), what is the suggested number of servings ((for example ½ cup of cooked? rice = 1 serving) of carbohydrates per day for a 2,000 calorie diet? (circle one)
    A. 4 servings
    B. 6 servings
    C. 8 servings
    D. 10 servings

26. How many teaspoons are in one tablespoon? (circle one)
    A. 2 teaspoons
    B. 3 teaspoons
    C. 4 teaspoons

27. Which of these is not a recommended serving size of protein foods? (circle one)
    A. A 3-ounce piece of fish
    B. Two scrambled eggs
    C. ¼ cup of hummus
    D. A 3-ounce steak

28. Which of these portion sizes of vegetables, proteins, and starchy foods would be the most helpful for weight loss? (circle one)

A. 1/2 plate vegetables, 1/4 protein, 1/4 whole-grain starches
B. 1/4 the plate vegetables, 1/2 protein, 1/4 whole-grain starches
C. 1/3 plate vegetables, 1/3 protein, 1/3 whole-grain starches
D. 1/4 the plate vegetables, 1/4 protein, 1/2 whole-grain starches

29. How large is a 3 ounce piece of chicken? (circle one)
   A. Size of a baseball
   B. Size of a deck of cards
   C. Size of small box of matches
   D. Size of a brick

30. How many fluid ounces are in one cup? (circle one)
   A. 8
   B. 10
   C. 12
   D. 14

31. You are following a diet that includes one serving of diary for breakfast.
   Which of the following choices would be appropriate? (circle one)
   A. 2 cups of whole milk
   B. 4 ounces of cheddar cheese
   C. 1 cup of cottage cheese
   D. 2/3 cup of unsweetened yogurt

32. Which of these portion sizes of granola cereal and corn flake cereal would
   be the most helpful for weight loss?
   A. 1 cup granola and 1 cup corn flake cereal
   B. 1 cup granola and ½ cup corn flake cereal
   C. ½ cup granola and 1 cup corn flake cereal
   D. 1 cup granola and 2 cups corn flake cereal

33. You are trying to control your weight by follow a meal plan that includes
   one serving of vegetables and one serving of fat for lunch. Which of the
   following choices would be appropriate? (circle one)
   A. One cup of cooked carrots with two teaspoons of regular mayonnaise
   B. Two cups of zucchini with 14 almonds
   C. two cup of asparagus and 2 pats of butter
   D. Two cups of spinach with 2 teaspoons of ranch dressing

34. You are following a diet that includes one serving of fruit for a snack.
   Which of the following choices would be appropriate? (circle one)
   A. ½ cup of whole strawberries
   B. One cup of unsweetened 100% orange juice

C. One banana

D. 40 whole cherries

35. You are following a diet that includes two serving of protein and two
serving of carbohydrates for dinner. Which of the following choices would
be appropriate? (circle one)
A. 4-ounces of cooked lean hamburger on a 2 small whole-grain bun
B. 12-ounces of grilled fish and 2 cup of cooked brown rice
C. 2 small smoked sausage links with 2 whole grain bagel
D. 5-ounces of cooked skinless chicken with 2 cups of whole-grain
cooked pasta

36. How large is one serving of fruit? (circle one)
A. The size of one dice
B. The size of one ping pong ball
A. The size one tennis ball
B. The size of two tennis balls

37. Which of these food groups is recommended by the United States
Department of Agriculture (USDA) for a healthy diet?

Fruits & Vegetables
Protein
Water
Grains
Dairy

A.

Fruits
Grains
Dairy
Vegetables
Protein

B.

Fruits
Protein
Dairy
Vegetables
Grains

C.

Grains
Dairy
Water
Vegetables & Fruits
Protein

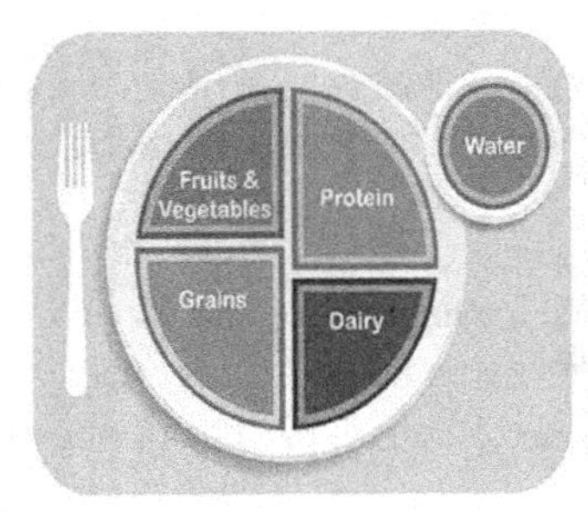

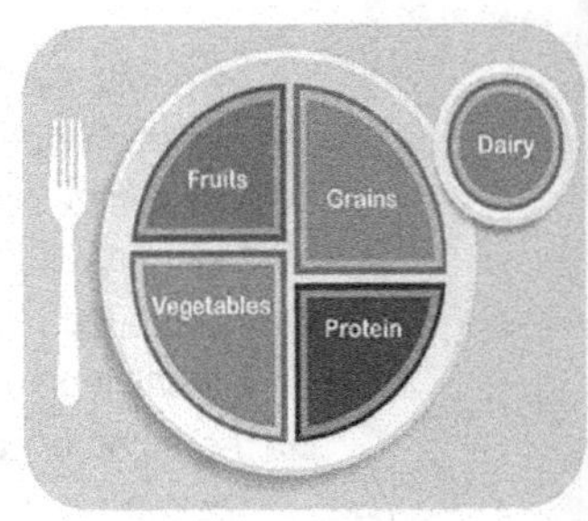

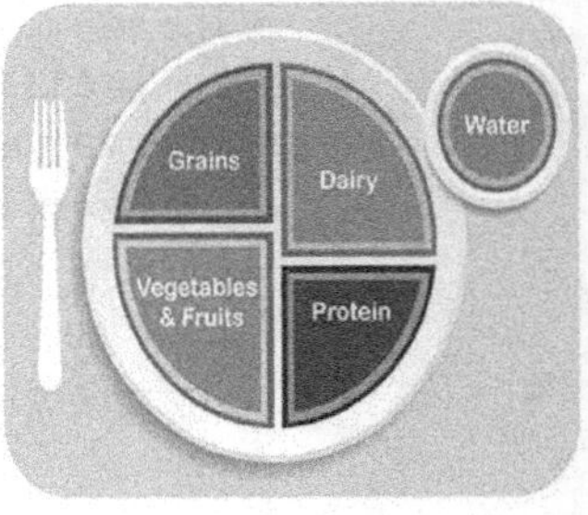

D.

Section E: Effect of alcohol intake

38. Wine and beer are low in calories: (circle one)
    A. True
    B. False

39. Alcohol alone has no calories, but it is bad for your health: (circle one)
    A. True
    B. False

40. Which of the following has more calories? (circle one)
    A. One cup of beer 4% alcohol
    B. One cup of wine 12.5% alcohol
    C. One cup of whisky 43.0% alcohol
    D. All of the above have similar amount of calories

41. Which of the following is true:
    A. Alcoholic beverages can reduce your appetite
    B. Alcoholic beverages can increase your appetite
    C. Alcoholic beverages have no effect on your appetite

Section F: How to identify needed nutrition information from a variant of sources

42. If you drink the entire bottle of energy drink that has this label; how many calories did you consume? (circle one)

Nutrition Facts

Serving Size 3/4 cups (55g)

Servings Per Container 5

Amount Per Serving

Calories 250   Calories from Fat 50

	% Daily Values*
Total Fat 6g	**9%**
Saturated Fat 0.5g	**3%**
Trans Fat 0g	
Sodium 200mg	**8%**
Total Carbohydrate 40g	**13%**
Dietary Fiber 4g	**16%**
Sugars 18g	
Protein 9g	**18%**

*Percent Daily Values are based on a 2,000 calorie diet.

A. 250 calories
B. 275 calories
C. 1,250 calories
D. 2,000 calories

43. How many calories would you consume if you ate this whole bag of chips? (circle one)

<table>
<tr><td colspan="2">

Nutrition Facts

Serving Size 1 oz (28g)
</td></tr>
<tr><td colspan="2">**Amount Per Serving**</td></tr>
<tr><td>**Calories** 150</td><td>Calories from Fat 70</td></tr>
<tr><td></td><td>% Daily Values*</td></tr>
<tr><td>**Total Fat** 8g</td><td>12%</td></tr>
<tr><td>Saturated Fat 1g</td><td>5%</td></tr>
<tr><td>Trans Fat 0g</td><td></td></tr>
<tr><td>**Sodium** 180mg</td><td>8%</td></tr>
<tr><td>**Total Carbohydrate** 18g</td><td>6%</td></tr>
<tr><td>Dietary Fiber 2g</td><td>8%</td></tr>
<tr><td>Sugars 0g</td><td></td></tr>
<tr><td>**Protein** 2g</td><td>4%</td></tr>
<tr><td colspan="2">*Percent Daily Values are based on a 2,000 calorie diet.</td></tr>
</table>

A. 150 calories
B. 336 calories
C. 450 calories
D. Cannot be determine from the information given

44. Which information is not included on the Nutrition Facts panel of a food label?
A. The number of servings in the container
B. The calories in a serving of the food
C. The serving size of the food
D. The appropriate portion size of the food

45. Which of these indicates that a loaf of bread contains whole grains?
    A. The front of the package says "wheat"
    B. The bread is brown in color
    C. The fiber content is 5 grams or more per serving
    D. The words "whole grain" or "whole wheat" are among the first 3
        ingredients listed
    E. The bread is located in the organic section of the grocery store

46. How many calories would you consume if you drink one cup of this juice?
    (circle one)

Nutrition Facts

Serving Size 3/4 cups (55g)
Servings Per Container 5

Amount Per Serving

Calories 250   Calories from Fat 50

	% Daily Values*
Total Fat 6g	9%
Saturated Fat 0.5g	3%
Trans Fat 0g	
Sodium 200mg	8%
Total Carbohydrate 40g	13%
Dietary Fiber 4g	16%
Sugars 18g	
Protein 9g	18%

*Percent Daily Values are based on a 2,000 calorie diet.

    A. 200 calories
    B. 250 calories
    C. 330 calories
    D. 1,250 calories

47. You have decided that for breakfast you will eat a single, standard size cup of yogurt in the morning. When trying to choose between two types of yogurt, which one is better for weight loss? (circle one)

A)

Nutrition Facts	
Serving Size 1 container (300g)	
Servings Per Container 1	
Amount Per Serving	
Calories 150	Calories from Fat 35
	% Daily Values*
Total Fat 4g	6%
Saturated Fat 3g	15%
Trans Fat 0g	
Cholesterol 10mg	3%
Sodium 65mg	3%
Total Carbohydrate 8g	3%
Dietary Fiber 0g	0%
Sugars 8g	
Protein 20g	40%
*Percent Daily Values are based on a 2,000 calorie diet.	

B)

Nutrition Facts	
Serving Size 1 container (150g)	
Servings Per Container 1	
Amount Per Serving	
Calories 140	Calories from Fat 15
	% Daily Values*
Total Fat 1.5g	2%
Saturated Fat 1g	5%
Trans Fat 0g	
Cholesterol 5mg	2%
Sodium 85mg	4%
Total Carbohydrate 26g	9%
Dietary Fiber 0g	0%
Sugars 24g	
Protein 6g	12%
*Percent Daily Values are based on a 2,000 calorie diet.	

A. Eating one cup of yogurt from food label A
B. Eating one cup of yogurt from food label B

48. What characteristics of web-based information make it more likely to be reliable? (circle all that applies)
   A. The website is a government website with .gov in the search title
   B. The website is from a university or established medical centers
   C. The website includes many endorsements from real people
   D. The website promises good results or you money back

49. What characteristics of web-based weight management information make it less likely to be reliable? (circle all that applies)
   A. The website offers to sell you the product for weight loss at a discount
   B. The website provides information that is so advanced no one else has done it before
   C. The website provides weight management information that summarizes the research that has already been published
   D. The information is about a product that is sponsored by a well-known celebrity

APPENDIX 2

50. Which of the following single, standard size cups of yogurt for breakfast would be a better choice for weight loss? (circle one answer)

B)

Nutrition Facts	
Serving Size 1 container (300g)	
Servings Per Container 1	
Amount Per Serving	
Calories 140	Calories from Fat 35
	% Daily Values*
Total Fat 4g	6%
Saturated Fat 3g	15%
Trans Fat 0g	
Cholesterol 10mg	3%
Sodium 65mg	3%
Total Carbohydrate 8g	3%
Dietary Fiber 0g	0%
Sugars 6g	
Protein 20g	40%
*Percent Daily Values are based on a 2,000 calorie diet.	

B)

Nutrition Facts	
Serving Size 1 container (150g)	
Servings Per Container 1	
Amount Per Serving	
Calories 140	Calories from Fat 15
	% Daily Values*
Total Fat 1.5g	2%
Saturated Fat 1g	5%
Trans Fat 0g	
Cholesterol 5mg	2%
Sodium 85mg	4%
Total Carbohydrate 26g	9%
Dietary Fiber 0g	0%
Sugars 24g	
Protein 6g	12%
*Percent Daily Values are based on a 2,000 calorie diet.	

C. Eating one cup of yogurt with food label A
D. Eating one cup of yogurt with food label B

51. When cooking a quart of mixed dish (casserole) with beef, adding 2 cups of vegetables would: (select one answer)
D. Increase the amount of calories per 1 cup
E. Decrease the amount of calories per 1 cup
F. Not change the amount of calories per 1 cup

52. Which of the following statements indicates that a loaf of bread contains whole grains? (circle one answer)
F. The front of the package says "wheat"
G. The bread is brown in color
H. The fiber content is 2 grams or more per serving
I. The words "whole grain" or "whole wheat" are among the first 3 ingredients listed
J. The bread is located in the organic section of the grocery store

53. How does eating a greater proportion of foods like fruits, beans, and vegetables help people lose weight? (select one answer)
    E. They contain a lot of water
    F. They contain a lot of fiber
    G. Both A and B are correct
    H. They contain vitamins and antioxidants that help you lose weight

54. A 3-ounce portion of cooked meat is about the size of (select one answer)
    E. A baseball
    F. A small box of matches
    G. A brick
    H. A deck of cards

55. If you are working to lose weight and are on vacation where two different breakfast buffet styles are available. **Buffet A** offers a variety of fruits and whole grain bakeries. **Buffet B** offers a variety of fruits, pastries, dairy products, deli meats, and whole grain bakeries. Which choice will make it easier to keep your calorie intake lower? (select one answer)
    D. Pick Buffet A
    E. Pick Buffet B
    F. It doesn't matter which buffet because you'll eat the same amount of food

56. Which of the following contain fewer than 10 Calories? (select all that apply)
    F. Freshly brewed coffee with no sugar or milk
    G. Peach flavored herbal tea with no sugar added
    H. Freshly brewed tea with no sugar added
    I. Cranberry juice
    J. Skim milk

57. What characteristics of web-based nutrition information make it more likely to be reliable? (circle all that apply)
    A. The website is a government website with .gov in the search title
    B. The website is from a university or an established medical center
    C. The website includes many testimonials from people who lost weight
    D. The website promises good results or your money back

58. If someone ate the entire contents of this package, how many Calories would they consume? (select one answer)

Nutrition Facts

Serving Size 3/4 cups (55g)
Servings Per Container 5

Amount Per Serving

Calories 250   Calories from Fat 50

	% Daily Values*
Total Fat 6g	**9%**
Saturated Fat 0.5g	**3%**
Trans Fat 0g	
Sodium 200mg	**8%**
Total Carbohydrate 40g	**13%**
Dietary Fiber 4g	**16%**
Sugars 18g	
Protein 9g	**18%**

*Percent Daily Values are based on a 2,000 calorie diet.

E. 250 Calories
F. 500 Calories
G. 1,250 Calories
H. 2,000 Calories

59. Which of these has the fewest calories? (select one answer)
E. Organic orange juice
F. Diet Cola
G. Gatorade
H. Skim milk

60. If you ate a half cup of each of these foods, which would have the most
    calories? (select one answer)
    E. Table sugar
    F. Starchy foods (potato, bread)
    G. Foods with lots of fiber (lettuce and broccoli)
    H. Fat (butter, cooking oil)

61. Do you think raspberries contain fiber?
    A. Yes
    B. No

62. Do you think Bananas contain fiber?
    A. Yes
    B. No

63. Do you think Eggs contain fiber?
    A. Yes
    B. No

64. Do you think red meats contain fiber?
    A. Yes
    B. No

65. Do you think broccoli contain fiber?
    A. Yes
    B. No

66. Do you think green peas contain fiber?
    A. Yes
    B. No

67. Do you think lentils/beans contain fiber?
    A. Yes
    B. No

68. Do you think fish contain fiber
    A. Yes
    B. No

69. Do you think artichoke contain fiber
    A. Yes
    B. No

70. Which of the following food servings has the fewest calories? (select one
    answer)
    E. 2 cups of raw spinach
    F. 2 tablespoons of olive oil
    G. 2 hardboiled eggs
    H. 2 thin slices of whole wheat bread

71. Health experts recommend that eating more servings of red meats (beef,
    pork, lamb, etc.) can be helpful as part of a diet to help reduce body fat.
    (select one answer)
    A. True
    B. False

72. If someone is trying to lose weight it is helpful that they add a cup of fresh
    orange juice with each meal: (select one answer)
    A. True
    B. False

73. According to the United States Department of Agriculture (USDA), a
    typical, normal weight woman needs about how many Calories per day to
    maintain her weight? (select one answer)
    E. 1,000 - 1,400 Calories
    F. 1,800- 2,200 Calories
    G. 2,400- 2,800 Calories
    H. 3,000- 3,400 Calories

74. Which of these is too large of a serving size for a protein food? (select one
    answer)
    E. A 3-ounce piece of fish
    F. 3 scrambled eggs
    G. ¼ cup of hummus
    H. A 3-ounce steak

75. Which of these meals with vegetables, meat, and starchy foods would be the most helpful for weight loss? (select one answer)
   E. 1/2 plate vegetables, 1/4 plate meat, 1/4 plate whole-grain starches
   F. 1/4 plate vegetables, 1/2 plate meat, 1/4 whole-grain starches
   G. 1/4 plate vegetables, 1/4 plate meat, ½ plate whole-grain starches

76. How many fluid ounces are in one cup? (select one answer)
   E. 8
   F. 10
   G. 12
   H. 14

77. Which of these is a good strategy to help to lose weight? (select one answer)
   D. Having a small number (<3) of foods to choose from per meal
   E. Having an average number (about 5) of foods to choose from per meal
   F. Having a large number (>7) foods to choose from per meal

78. Which of the following is the best choice for a weight control diet that includes one serving of dairy for breakfast? (select one answer)
   E. 2 cups of whole milk
   F. 4 ounces of cheddar cheese
   G. 1 cup of cottage cheese
   H. 1 cup of unsweetened yogurt

79. What does the term "calorie-dense foods" mean? (select one answer)
   D. Foods that have a lot of calories within smaller portions
   E. Foods that weigh more
   F. Foods that you have to eat a lot of to get enough calories

80. If served 100 calories of each of these foods, which would have the largest portion size? (select one answer)
   E. 1% fat cottage cheese
   F. Roasted chicken breast with the skin removed
   G. Regular (non-cream) tomato soup
   H. Bagel

81. How large is one medium apple or orange? (select one answer)
   C. The size of one dice
   D. The size of one ping pong ball
   E. The size of a tennis ball
   F. The size of a softball

82. Which of these food groups is recommended by the United States
   Department of Agriculture (USDA) for a healthy diet? (select one answer)

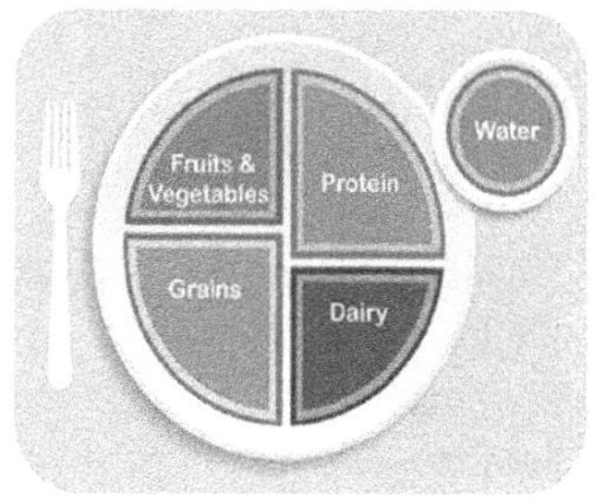

A.

B.

C.

D.

   A.
   B.
   C.
   D.

83. Which of the following has more calories? (select one answer)
   A. 8 ounces of beer 4% alcohol
   B. 8 ounces of wine 12.5% alcohol
   C. 8 ounces of whiskey 43.0% alcohol

D. All of the above have a similar amount of calories

84. Health experts recommend that eating more servings of foods high in starch (bread, potatoes, rice, etc.) can be helpful as part of a diet to help reduce body fat. (select one answer)
   A. True
   B. False

85. Which of the following has the fewest calories? (select one answer)
   E. 2 cups of vegetable beef stew
   F. 2 cups of vegetable beef soup
   G. 2 cups of vegetable beef lasagna
   H. They are all the same

86. All of the following information is included on the Nutrition Facts panel of a food label except (select one answer)
   E. The number of servings in the container
   F. The calories in a serving of the food
   G. The serving size of the food
   H. The amount to eat at a meal

87. How many Calories would someone get if they drank 1 1/2 cups of this beverage? (select one answer)

Nutrition Facts

Serving Size 3/4 cups (55g)
Servings Per Container 5

Amount Per Serving

Calories 250   Calories from Fat 50

	% Daily Values*
Total Fat 6g	**9%**
Saturated Fat 0.5g	**3%**
Trans Fat 0g	
Sodium 200mg	**8%**
Total Carbohydrate 40g	**13%**
Dietary Fiber 4g	**16%**
Sugars 18g	
Protein 9g	**18%**

*Percent Daily Values are based on a 2,000 calorie diet.

  E. 250 Calories
  F. 330 Calories
  G. 500 Calories
  H. 1,250 Calories

88. According to the United States Department of Agriculture (USDA), a typical, normal weight man needs about how many Calories per day to maintain his weight? (select one answer)
  E. 1,200- 1,600 Calories
  F. 1,800- 2,200 Calories
  G. 2,400- 2,800 Calories
  H. 3,000- 3,400 Calories

89. Which of these has the fewest calories? (select one answer)
  D. 1 cup of apple juice
  E. 1 can of regular (non-diet) soda
  F. 1 cup of orange juice
  G. 1 cup of skimmed milk

90. If each of these meals has the same calories, which would be the best choice for a low fat, high fiber meal? (select one answer)
  E. Grilled chicken with raspberry glaze
  F. Cheese on whole wheat toast

G. Beans on brown rice
H. Greek yogurt with honey

91. Health experts would consider wine and beer to be low-calorie beverages.
(select one answer)
C. True
D. False

92. Which of these strategies should help decrease the amount of calories
someone eats for a meal? (select one answer)
A. Choosing smaller portions of each food
B. Drinking a lot of water during a meal
C. Eating more spicy foods
D. Eating quickly

Nutrition Education Curriculum driven from the Look AHEAD Trial

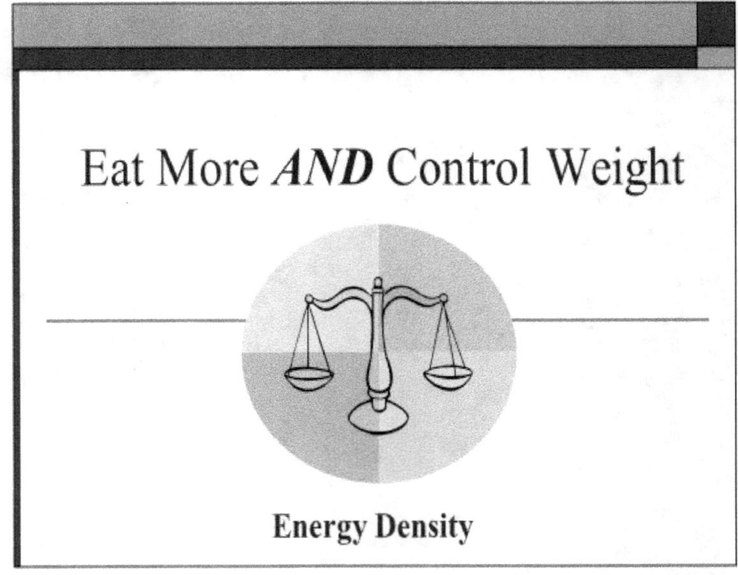

Objectives

- Define the concept of energy density
- Identify what nutrients lower energy density
- Explain how foods with low energy density help with weight loss
- Compare foods based on energy density

Key Points

- For many, feeling *full* is based on the *volume/weight* of a food- not on the calories consumed

- How can one eat *more volume* of food *without* increasing Calories?

Choose foods with

LOW ENERGY (Calorie) DENSITY

Low Energy (Calorie) Dense Foods

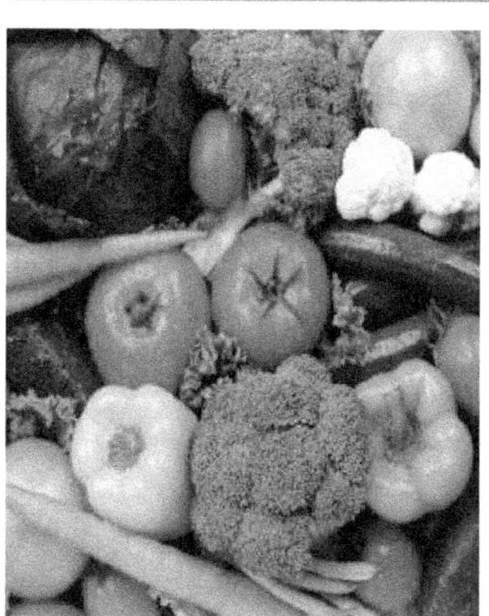

Foods with a **high water** and **fiber** content are **low** in **energy density** …
there are few calories per amount of food

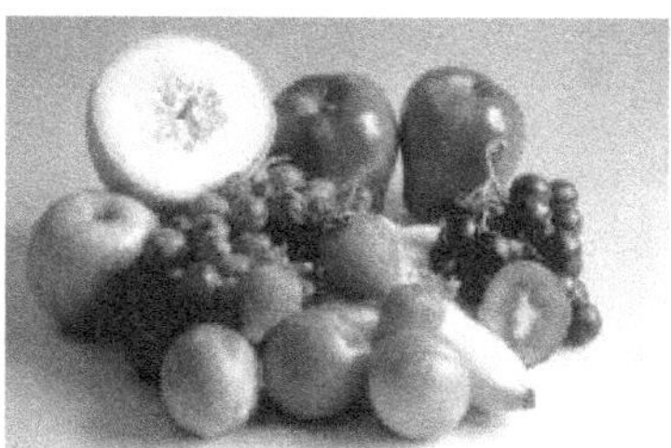

Energy (Calorie)Density

Simply Stated:
Number of Calories in a specific
amount or weight of food

Equation:
Energy Density = Calories/gram

High Energy (Calorie) Dense Foods

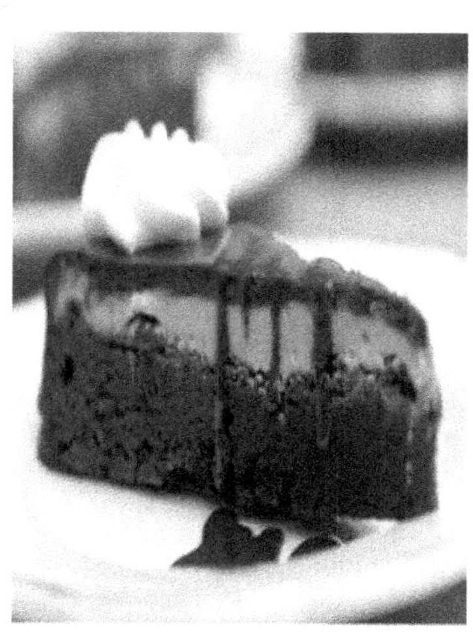

Foods **HIGH** in **fat,**
LOW in **water,** and
LOW in **fiber** are
HIGH in **energy density**…
there are more calories in a
small amount of food

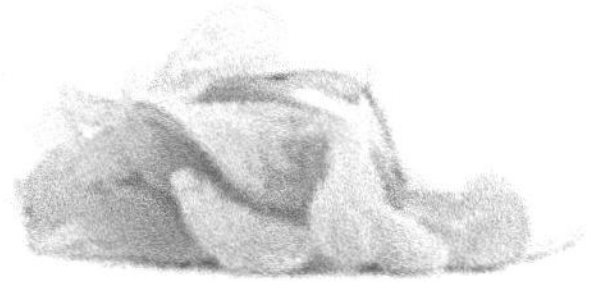

Energy (Calorie)Density

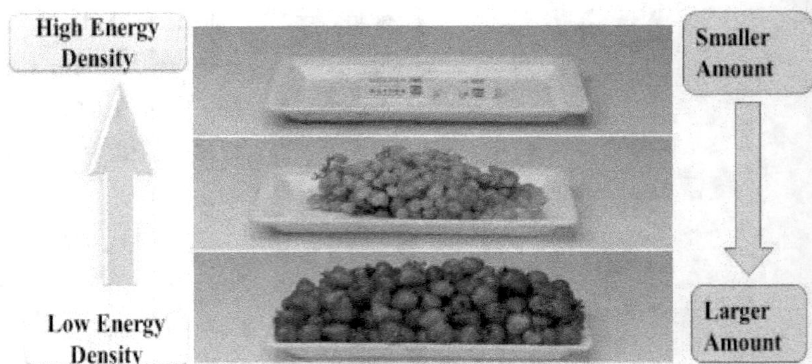

Each platter of food provides 1200 Calories

Nutrients that lower energy density:

Water

- Contains zero calories
- Has weight

Fiber

- *Minimal* calories
- Has weight

Water Content of Foods

Fruits and Vegetables	80-95%
Milk	87%
Meat	45-65%
Bread	35-45%
Oil	0

Finding Fiber…

Fiber found in foods from **PLANTS**

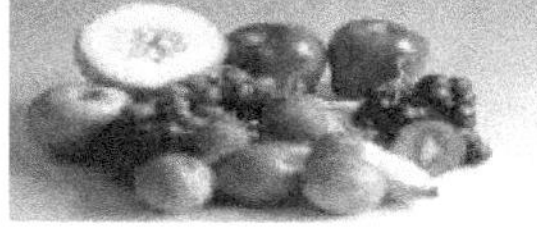

- Fruits and Vegetables
- Whole Grains/Starches
- Legumes – Beans, Lentils, Peas

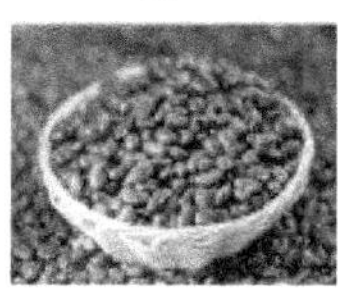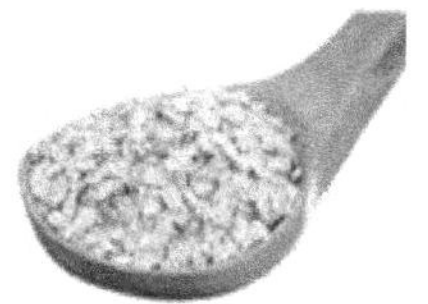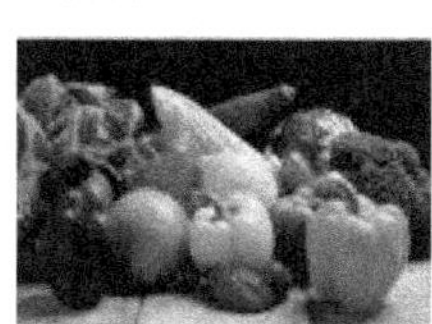

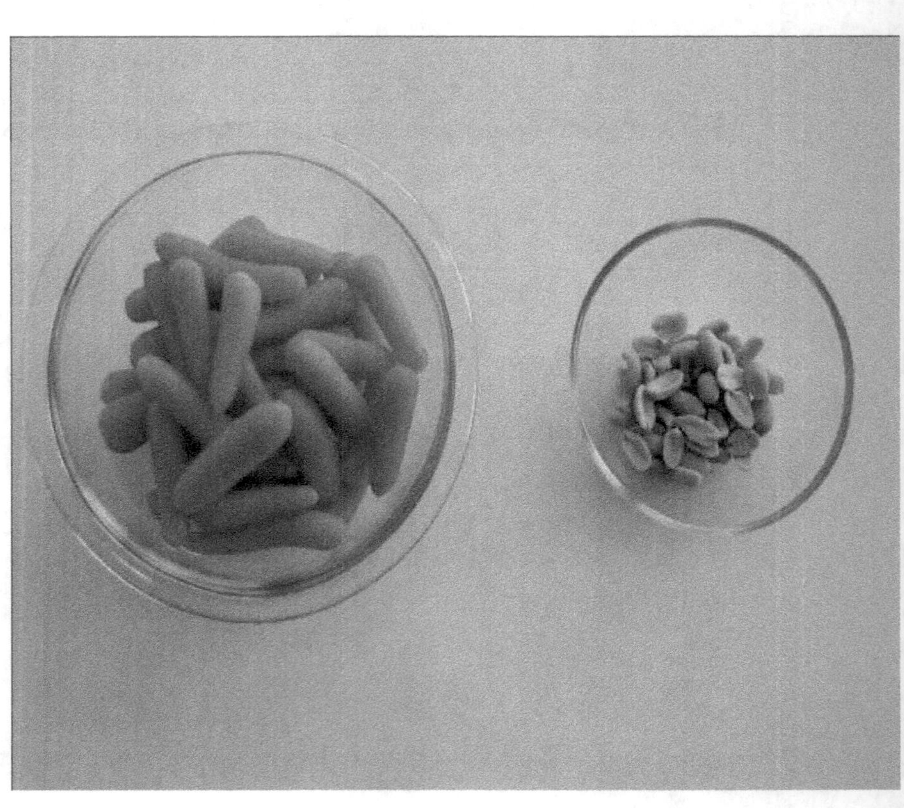

Energy (Calorie)Density Comparison of Foods

Carrots

Serving size: **428 grams (~2 cups)**

Calories: **168**

Fiber: 8.5 grams

Low energy density:

168 Calories/428 grams = 0.39 Calories/gram of food

Peanuts

Serving size: **28 grams (~0.11 cups   or   1 ounce)**

Calories: **170**

Fiber: 2 grams

High energy density:

170 Calories/28 grams = 6 Calories/gram of food

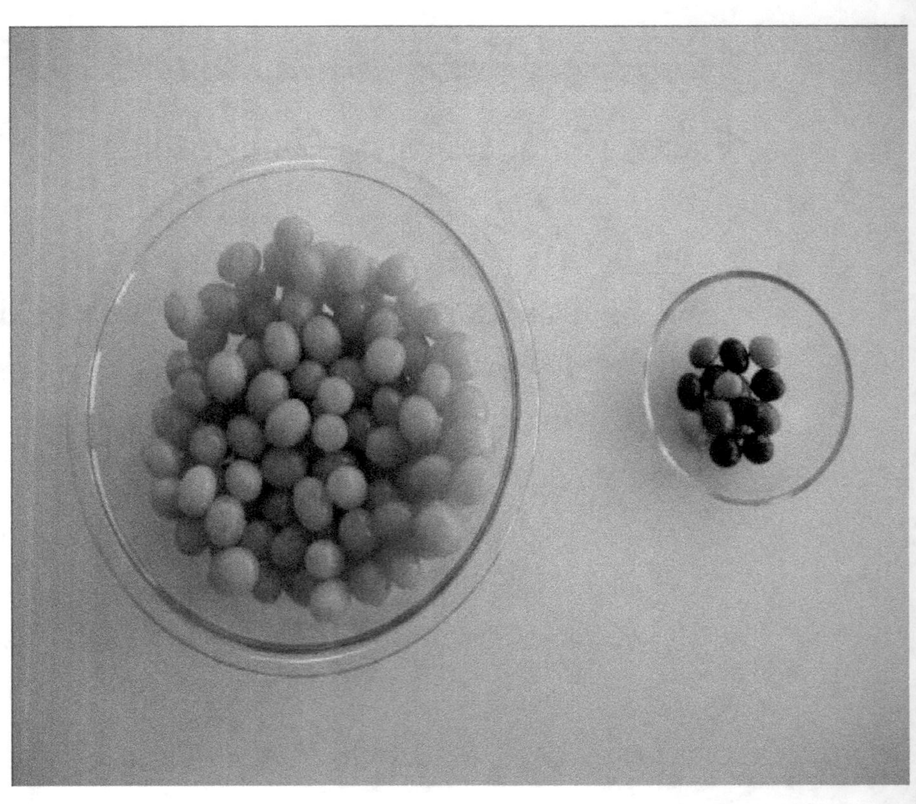

Even Air can Reduce Energy Density

Adding air to food = zero extra Calories
By making the serving bigger it is possible to
consume fewer calories with larger portion sizes

Examples of foods that are made larger by
adding air…

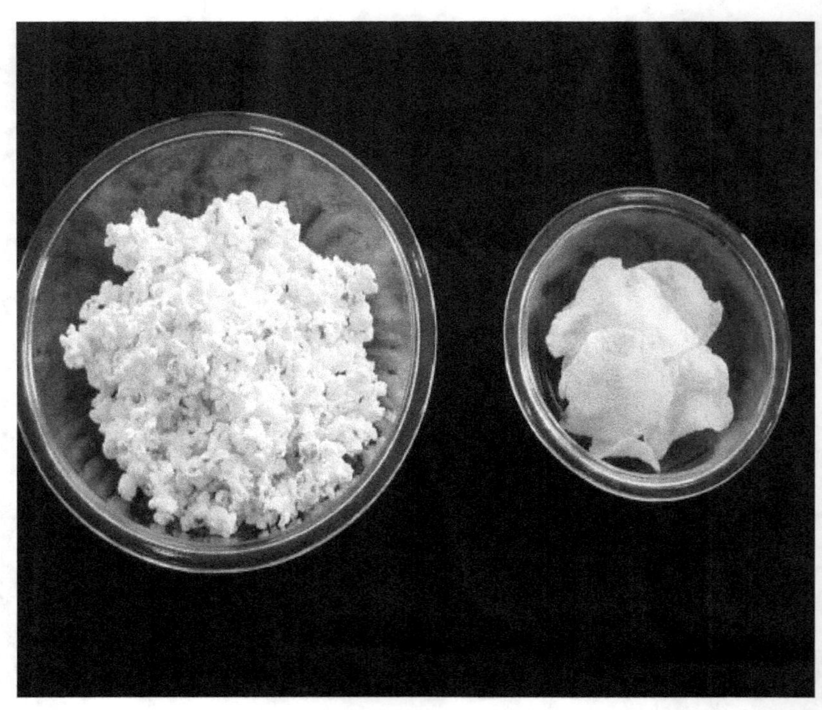

Class Activity:
Food Labels and Energy Density

Energy Density   = Calories/gram

Calculating Energy (Calorie) Density - *Simplified*

Calories < grams	Low energy density
Calories up to twice the grams	Medium energy density
Calories > twice the grams	High energy density

Activity: Labels and Energy(Calorie)Density

Recall: Energy Density = Calories < Grams = low energy density

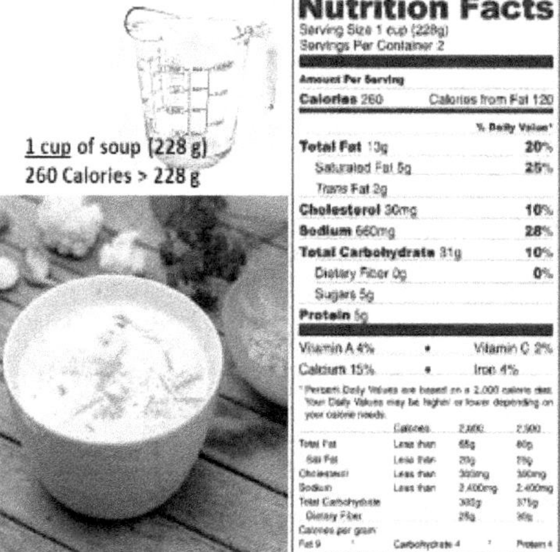

1 cup of soup (228 g)
260 Calories > 228 g

Cream/high fat soup

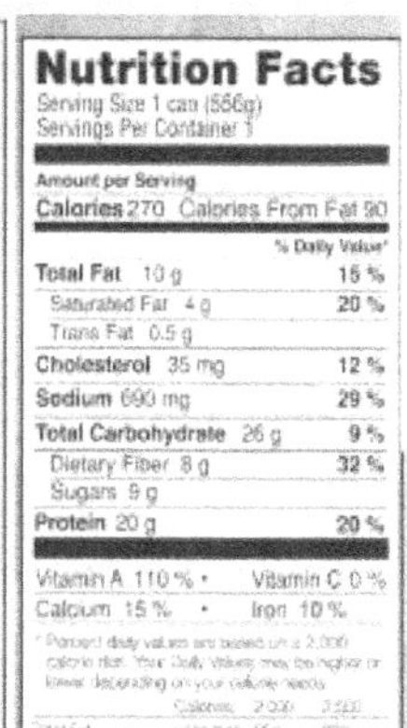

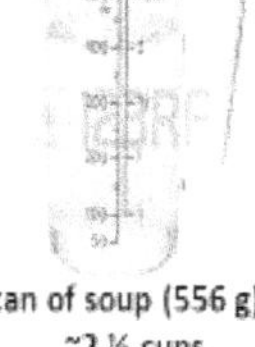

1 can of soup (556 g)
~2 ½ cups
270 Calories < 556 g
Low energy density

Broth based soup

Which soup provides a larger amount/volume for the same Calories?

Summary:
A lot of food for the same amount of Calories!

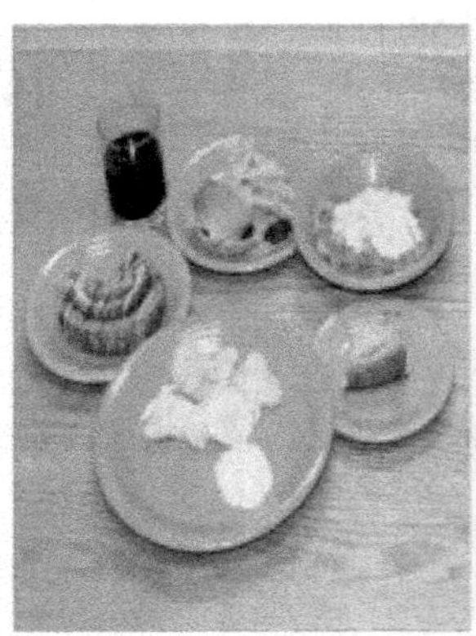

1575 Kcal
High Energy Density

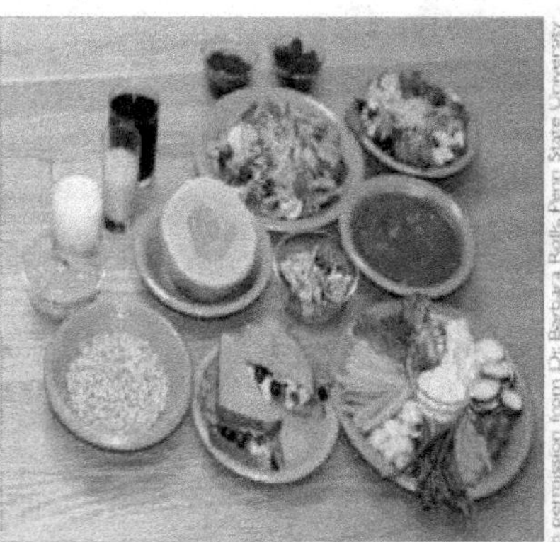

1575 Kcal
Low Energy Density

Nutrition Facts Label
Portion Control
Healthy Food Choices

Yogurt

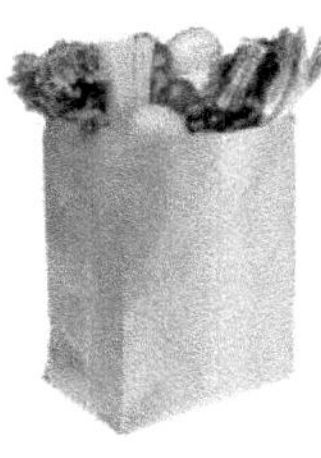
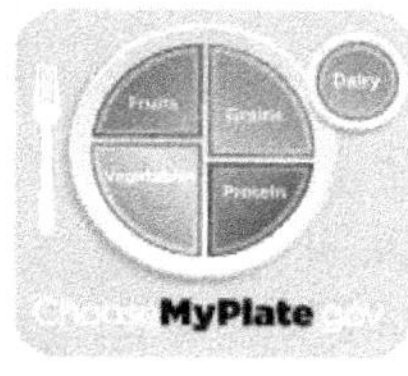

Nutrition Facts

Serving Size 1 container

Amount Per Serving

Calories 180 | Calories from Fat 23

% Daily Value*

Total Fat 2.5g | 4%

Saturated Fat 1.5g | 6%

Trans Fat 0g

Cholesterol 15mg | 4%

Sodium 110mg | 5%

Potassium 290mg | 8%

Total Carbohydrate 31g | 10%

Sugars 28g

Protein 7g

Vitamin A 15% | Vitamin D 20%

Calcium 30% | Phosphorus 20%

INGREDIENTS: CULTURED PASTEURIZED GRADE A REDUCED FAT MILK, SUGAR, NONFAT MILK, CONTAINS 2% OR LESS OF MODIFIED CORN STARCH, HIGH FRUCTOSE CORN SYRUP, KOSHER GELATIN, TRICALCIUM PHOSPHATE, COLORED WITH BEET JUICE CONCENTRATE, NATURAL FLAVOR, CITRIC ACID, VITAMIN A ACETATE, VITAMIN D.

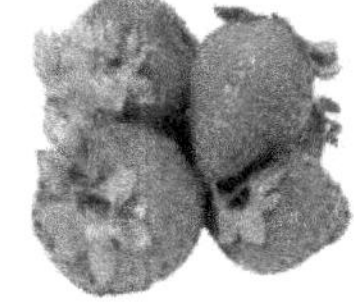

Objectives

* Understand how the volume, not the calories, of food is important in satisfying your hunger
* Identify key parts of a nutrition facts label
* Compare food labels for Calorie, nutrient, and serving information
* Define portion versus serving
* Use common items to identify serving sizes
* Describe the plate method for making healthy choices and controlling portions

* Do you currently look at the nutrition facts label when choosing a food or beverage?
* What do you look at on the label?
* What is confusing to you on the label?

Read the Nutrition Facts Label

Oatmeal

Nutrition Facts

Serving Size 1/2 cup dry (40g)
Servings Per Container About 30

Amount Per Serving

Calories 150	Calories from Fat 25

	% Daily Value*
Total Fat 3g	5%
Saturated Fat 0.5g	2%
Trans Fat 0g	
Polyunsaturated Fat 1g	
Monounsaturated Fat 1g	
Cholesterol 0mg	0%
Sodium 0mg	0%
Total Carbohydrate 27g	9%
Dietary Fiber 4g	16%
Soluble Fiber 2g	
Insoluble Fiber 2g	
Sugars 1g	
Protein 5g	

Vitamin A 0%	Vitamin C 0%
Calcium 0%	Iron 10%

*Percent Daily Values are based on a 2,000 calorie diet. Your daily values may be higher or lower depending on your calorie needs.

		Calories:	2,000	2,500
Total Fat	Less than		65g	80g
Sat Fat	Less than		20g	25g
Cholesterol	Less than		300mg	300mg
Sodium	Less than		2,400mg	2,400mg
Total Carbohydrate			300g	375g
Dietary Fiber			25g	30g

INGREDIENTS: 100% NATURAL WHOLE GRAIN ROLLED OATS

Serving Size

How many servings are in the container?

Calories in **one** serving

How many servings do you plan to eat?

How would this change the calories you consume?

Reading the
Nutrition Facts Label:

✓ Check the Serving Size
  - How many servings are in the container?
✓ Check the calories in one serving
  - How many servings do you plan to eat?
✓ Check the % Daily Value
  - 5% or less is low
    - Limit nutrients shown in orange
  - 20% or more is high
    - Get enough of nutrients shown in green

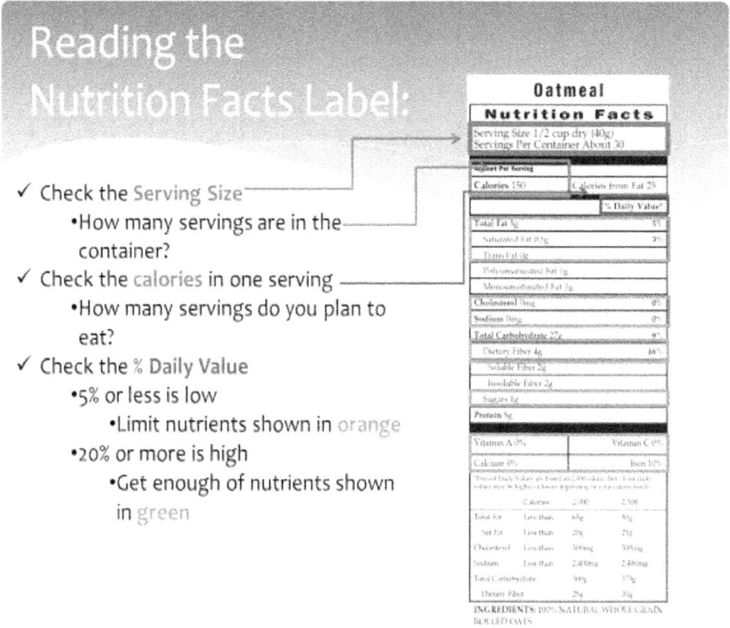

Check the Ingredients List

Whole Grains

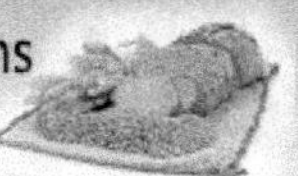

* Descending order by weight

* Ingredients listed from highest to lowest amounts by weight

    * **Tip:** Look at the *TOP THREE*

Whole Wheat Flour

INGREDIENTS: WHOLE WHEAT FLOUR (WHOLE GRAIN), CRACKED WHOLE WHEAT, WATER, BROWN SUGAR, WHEAT GLUTEN, YEAST, CANOLA OIL (NON-HYDROGENATED), SALT, RAISIN, JUICE CONCENTRATE

Wheat Flour

INGREDIENTS: ENRICHED FLOUR (WHEAT FLOUR, NIACIN, REDUCED IRON, THIAMIN MONONITRATE, RIBOFLAVIN, FOLIC ACID), SALT, CORN OIL, CORN SYRUP, AMMONIUM BICARBONATE, MALT EXTRACT, AND YEAST. **CONTAINS A WHEAT INGREDIENT.**

NO PRESERVATIVES.

Smart Shopping and Reading the Nutrition Facts Label

Compare similar products

Nonfat (Skim) Milk

Nutrition Facts

Serving Size 1 cup (236ml)
Servings Per Container About 16

Amount Per Serving

Calories 80	Calories from Fat 0

	% Daily Value*
Total Fat 0g	0%
Saturated Fat 0g	0%
Trans Fat 0g	
Cholesterol Less than 5mg	0%
Sodium 120mg	5%
Total Carbohydrate 11g	4%
Dietary Fiber 0g	0%
Sugars 11g	
Protein 9g	

Vitamin A 10%	Vitamin C 4%
Calcium 30%	Iron 0%
Vitamin D 25%	

*Percent Daily Values are based on 2,000 calorie diet. Your daily values may be higher or lower depending on your calorie needs

Reduced Fat (2%) Milk

Nutrition Facts

Serving Size 1 cup (236ml)
Servings Per Container About 16

Amount Per Serving

Calories 120	Calories from Fat 45

	% Daily Value*
Total Fat 5g	8%
Saturated Fat 3g	15%
Trans Fat 0g	
Cholesterol 20mg	7%
Sodium 120mg	5%
Total Carbohydrate 11g	4%
Dietary Fiber 0g	0%
Sugars 11g	
Protein 9g	

Vitamin A 10%	Vitamin C 4%
Calcium 30%	Iron 0%
Vitamin D 25%	

*Percent Daily Values are based on 2,000 calorie diet. Your daily values may be higher or lower depending on your calorie needs

Regular Chips

Nutrition Facts

Serving Size 1 oz. (28g / About 15 chips)
Servings Per Container About 11

Amount Per Serving

Calories 160	Calories from Fat 90

	% Daily Value*
Total Fat 10g	15%
Saturated Fat 1g	5%
Trans Fat 0g	
Polyunsaturated Fat 2.5g	
Monounsaturated Fat 5g	
Cholesterol 0mg	0%
Sodium 170mg	7%
Potassium 390mg	10%
Total Carbohydrate 15g	5%
Dietary Fiber 1g	5%
Sugars less than 1g	
Protein 2g	

Vitamin A 0%		Vitamin C 10%	
Calcium 0%		Iron 2%	
Vitamin E 6%		Thiamin 4%	
Niacin 6%		Vitamin B₆ 10%	
Magnesium 4%		Zinc 2%	

*Percent Daily Values are based on 2,000 calorie diet. Your daily values may be higher or lower depending on your calorie needs.

	Calories	2,000	2,500
Total Fat	Less than	65g	80g
Sat Fat	Less than	20g	25g
Cholesterol	Less than	300mg	300mg
Sodium	Less than	2,400mg	2,400mg
Potassium		3,500mg	3,500mg
Total Carbohydrate		300g	375g
Dietary Fiber		25g	30g

Calories per gram:
Fat 9 • Carbohydrate 4 • Protein 4

INGREDIENTS: POTATOES, VEGETABLE OIL (SUNFLOWER, CORN AND/OR CANOLA OIL) AND SALT. NO PRESERVATIVES

Baked Chips

Nutrition Facts

Serving Size 1 oz. (28g / About 15 chips)
Servings Per Container About 9

Amount Per Serving

Calories 120	Calories from Fat 20

	% Daily Value*
Total Fat 2g	3%
Saturated Fat 0g	0%
Trans Fat 0g	
Cholesterol 0mg	0%
Sodium 130mg	6%
Potassium 270mg	8%
Total Carbohydrate 23g	8%
Dietary Fiber 2g	8%
Sugars 2g	
Protein 2g	

Vitamin A 0%		Vitamin C 4%	
Calcium 0%		Iron 2%	
Thiamin 6%		Riboflavin 2%	
Niacin 6%		Vitamin B₆ 15%	
Phosphorus 4%		Magnesium 4%	

*Percent Daily Values are based on 2,000 calorie diet. Your daily values may be higher or lower depending on your calorie needs.

	Calories	2,000	2,500
Total Fat	Less than	65g	80g
Sat Fat	Less than	20g	25g
Cholesterol	Less than	300mg	300mg
Sodium	Less than	2,400mg	2,400mg
Potassium		3,500mg	3,500mg
Total Carbohydrate		300g	375g
Dietary Fiber		25g	30g

Calories per gram:
Fat 9 • Carbohydrate 4 • Protein 4

INGREDIENTS: DRIED POTATOES, CORN STARCH, SUGAR, CORN OIL, SALT, SOY LECITHIN, AND CORN SUGAR. **CONTAINS A SOY INGREDIENT.** NO PRESERVATIVES

Compare similar products

http://www.accessdata.fda.gov/videos/CFSAN/HWM/hwmintro.cfm

What Do You Need to Know?

- People eat roughly the same volume of food each day
- If you eat foods with many calories per bite you will likely consume more calories (example: higher fat choices)
- Foods with more fiber, water and air have fewer calories per bite – can eat larger amounts to help feel full without a lot of calories
- Large serving sizes will likely "drive" you to eat more than you *naturally* would eat

Portion Versus Serving

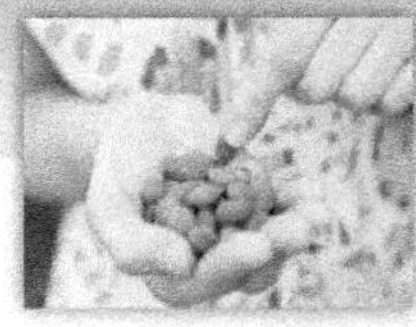

* **Portion** – the amount we actually eat
* **Serving** – a standard amount of a particular food

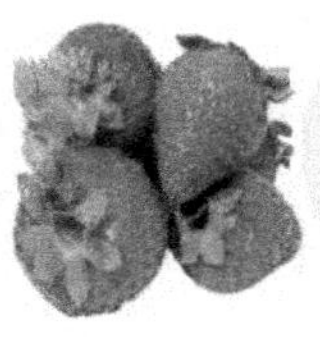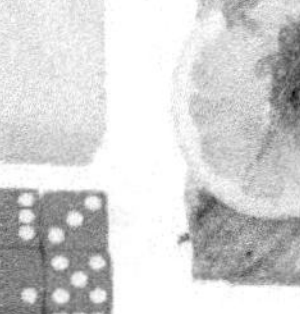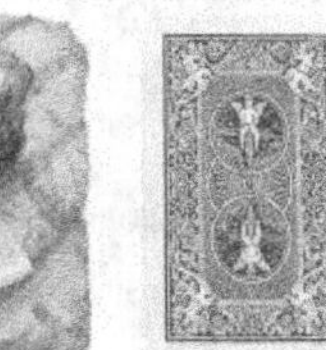

Visual Guide for Serving Size

How to count servings

Vegetables	Calories	Visual cue	
1 cup broccoli	25	1 baseball	
2 cups raw, leafy greens	25	2 baseballs	
Fruits	**Calories**	**Visual cue**	
½ cup sliced fruit	60	Tennis ball	
1 small apple or medium orange	60	Tennis ball	
Carbohydrates	**Calories**	**Visual cue**	
½ cup pasta or dry cereal	70	Hockey puck	
½ small bagel	70	Hockey puck	
1 slice whole-grain bread	70	Hockey puck	
½ medium baked potato	70	Hockey puck	
Protein/Dairy	**Calories**	**Visual cue**	
3 ounces of fish	110	Deck of cards	
2-2½ ounces of meat	110	⅔ deck of cards	
1½-2 ounces of hard cheese	110	⅓ deck of cards	
Fats	**Calories**	**Visual cue**	
1½ teaspoons peanut butter	45	2 dice	
1 teaspoon butter or margarine	45	1 die	

Healthy Choices: Use the Plate

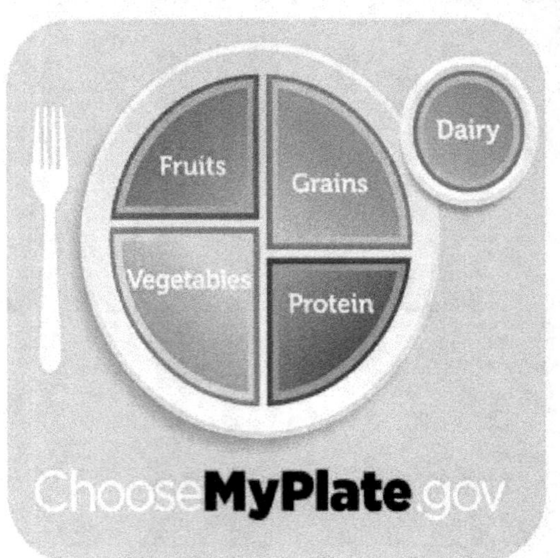

Focus on Fruits

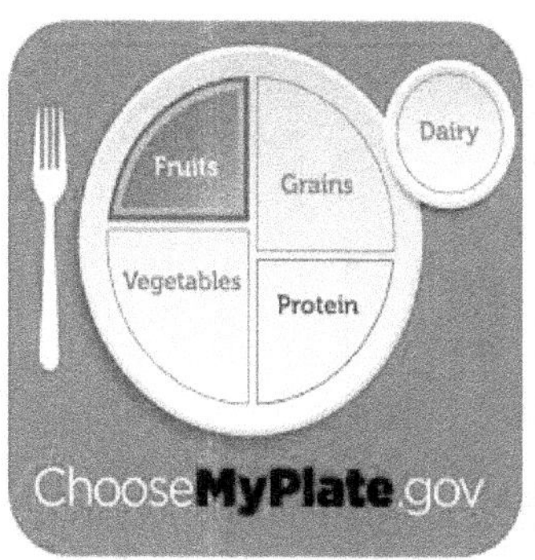

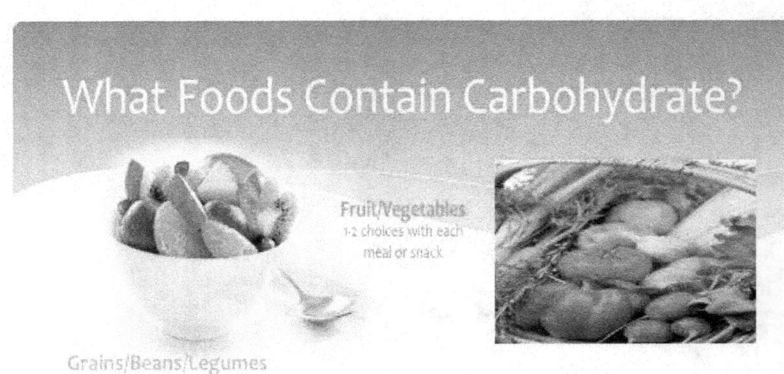

What Foods Contain Carbohydrate?
Fruit/Vegetables
1-2 choices with each
meal or snack

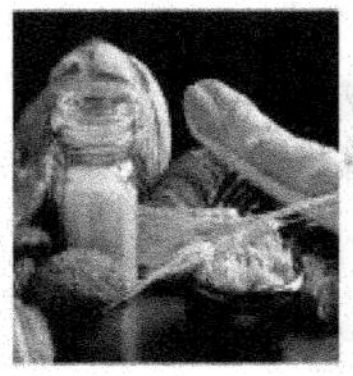
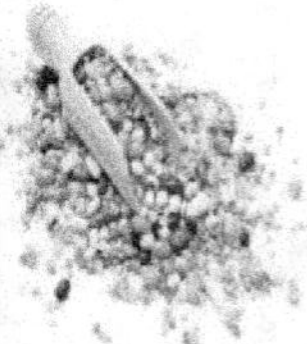

Grains/Beans/Legumes
Make at least half your grain choices
whole grains

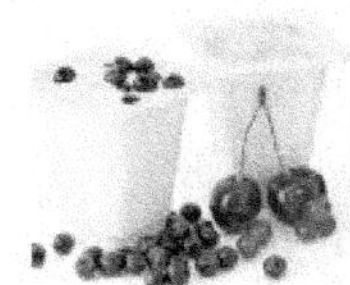

Dairy (Milk, Yogurt)
Choose low fat or fat-free
3 low-fat servings daily
1 cup milk
8 ounces yogurt

Protein-Rich Foods

- Fish
- Chicken, turkey
- Pork
- Lean beef
- Eggs
- Milk, yogurt, cheese
- Lentils, beans, tofu
- Nuts*

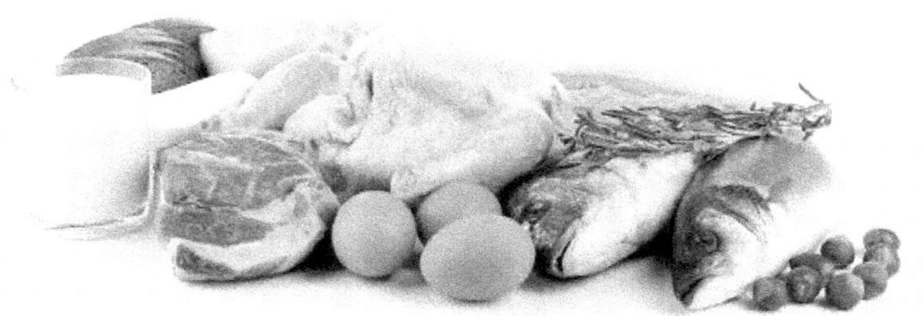

Choose Healthy Fats

* Most calorie dense at 9 calories per gram
  * One teaspoon is 5 grams of fat: 9 x 5= 45 calories

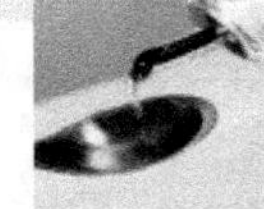

* Aim for 20 to 35% of daily calories

* Choose unsaturated fats more often than saturated fats (animal products, tropical oils*)

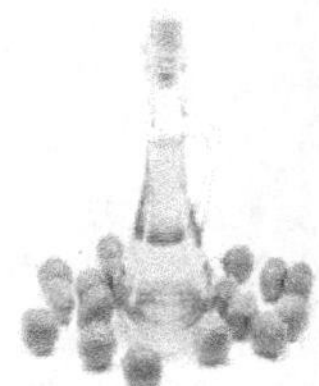

* Avoid trans fats – partially hydrogenated fats
* Bottom line:
  * All fats provide same amount of Calories!
  * To control Calories – moderate fat intake!

Flavoring Food Without Calories

Use Herbs and Spices

- Add lots of flavor with **negligible** calories
- Use in place of added fats (recipes, at meal times) to reduce calories

Flavoring	Amount	Calories
Salt	1 teaspoon	0
Basil	1 teaspoon	2
Cinnamon	1 teaspoon	2
Pepper	1 teaspoon	6
Oil, butter, margarine	1 teaspoon	45

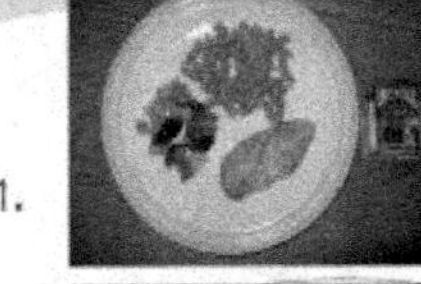

What about Calories and the Plate?
Which picture below is closest to 400 calories?

1.
278
calories

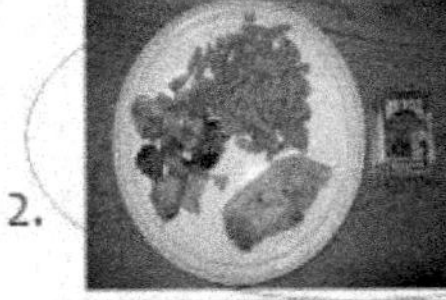

2.
447
calories

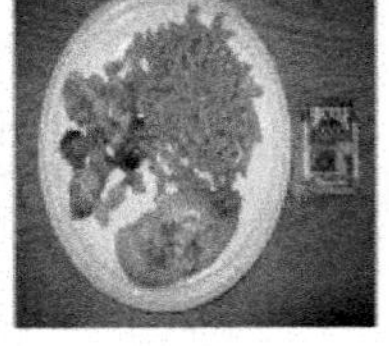

3.
616
calories

What is a daily Calorie recommendation?

What do you think the
recommendation is
for Men ?
for Women?

http://www.cnpp.usda.gov/sites/def
ault/files/usda_food_patterns/Estim
atedCalorieNeedsPerDayTable.pdf

Why Did You Choose It?

How Can You Consume Fewer Calories and Still be Satisfied?

* **Select** foods you like that have more fiber and water
* **Take** smaller portion sizes of foods that have a lot of calories per bite (ex: higher fat choices)
* **Use** smaller plates so the food on the plate appears much larger

BEVERAGES & BUFFETS

Objectives

- Recognize added sugars on Nutrition Label

- Build awareness of portion sizes and calorie composition of beverages

- Recognize the "buffet effect"

- Identify reliable electronic resources

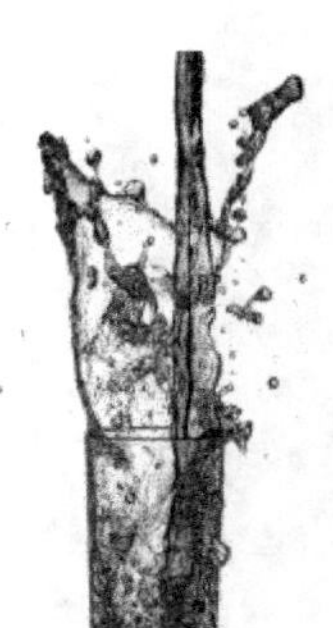

Sugar Sweetened Beverages

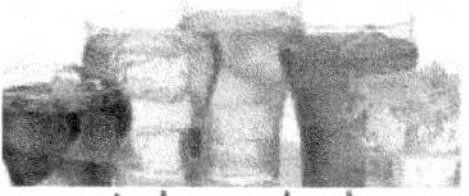

Sugar-sweetened beverages are those that contain caloric sweeteners and include:

- Soft drinks (soda pop)
- Fruit drinks
- Sports Drinks
- Sweet tea and flavored coffee drinks-
  - *Flavored* herbal teas can be naturally flavored (lemon, orange, etc...) and would **not** have calories)

https://www.caloriecount.com/calories-herbal-tea-ic1439

- Energy drinks
- Flavored milks or milk alternatives

Type of Milk	Serving: 1 cup = 8 ounces	Calories
Almond milk (unflavored)	8 oz.	60
(flavored – chocolate)	8 oz.	120
Skim milk (unflavored)	8 oz.	**90**
Soy milk (unflavored)	8 oz.	80
(flavored – chocolate)	8 oz.	120
Chocolate milk	8 oz.	158

Common Caloric Sweeteners

- High-fructose corn syrup
- Fructose
- Fruit juice concentrates
- Honey
- Sugar
- Syrup
- Corn syrup
- Sucrose
- Dextrose

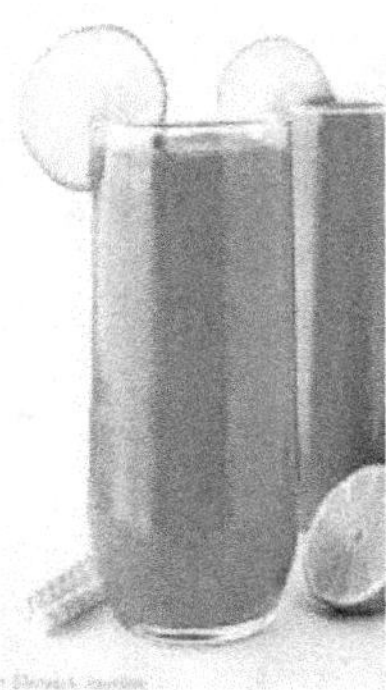

Reading Nutrition Facts Labels

Soda

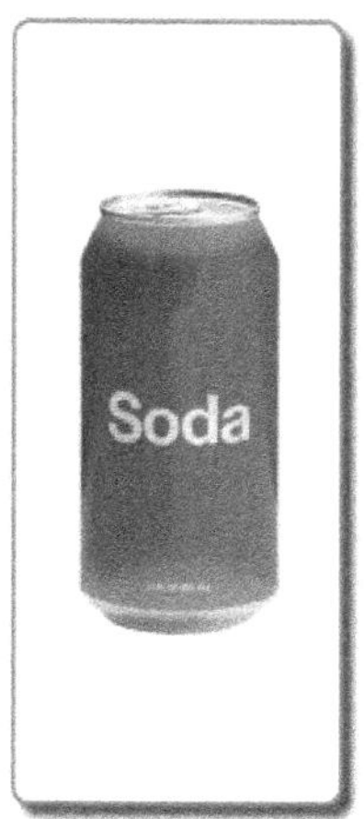

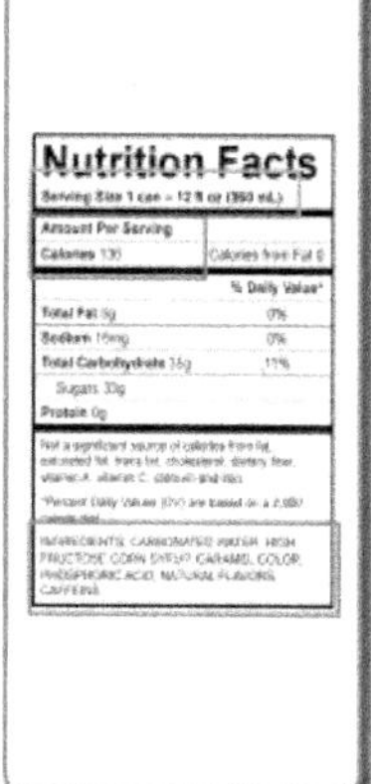

Serving Size

- How many servings in the container?

Calories in **one** serving

- How many servings do you plan to drink?

Check the ingredients

- Are there added sugars?

*** This material was produced by the California Department of Public Health's Network for a Healthy California with funding from USDA SNAP-Ed.

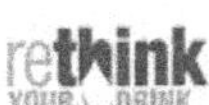

Juice Drink

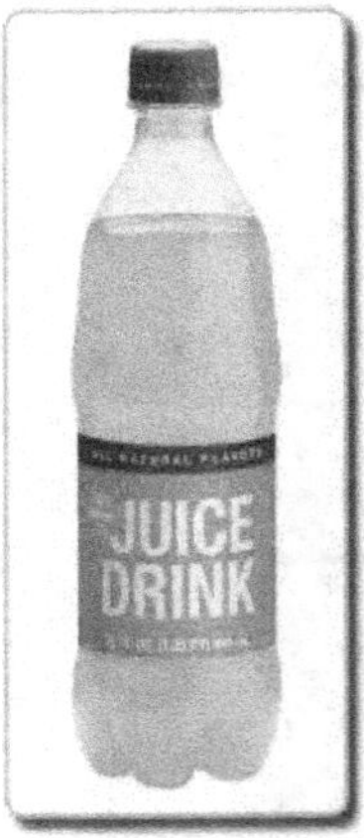

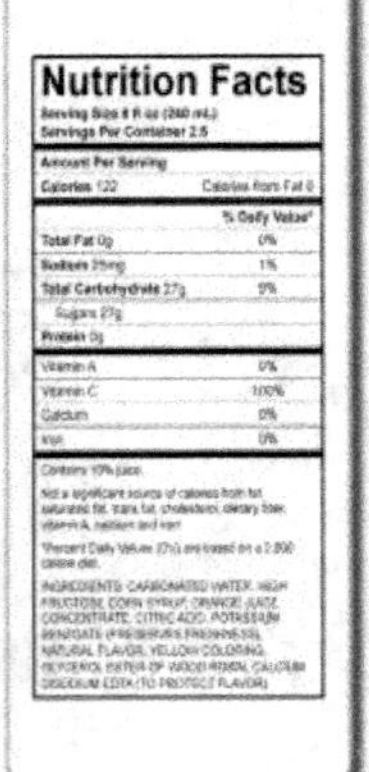

*** This material was produced by the California Department of Public Health's Network for a Healthy California with funding from USDA SNAP-Ed

Vitamin-added Water

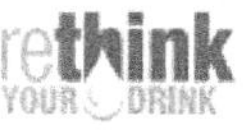

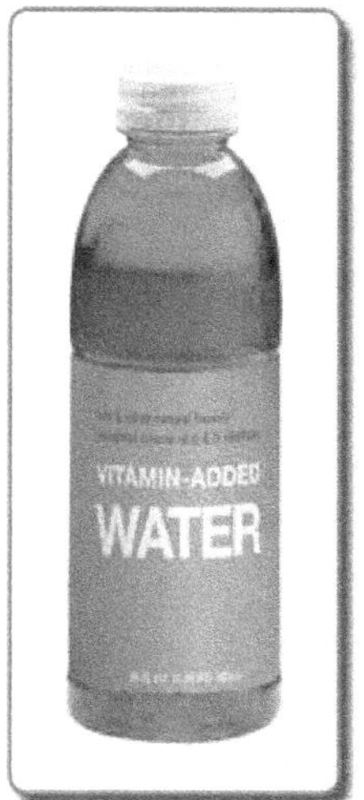

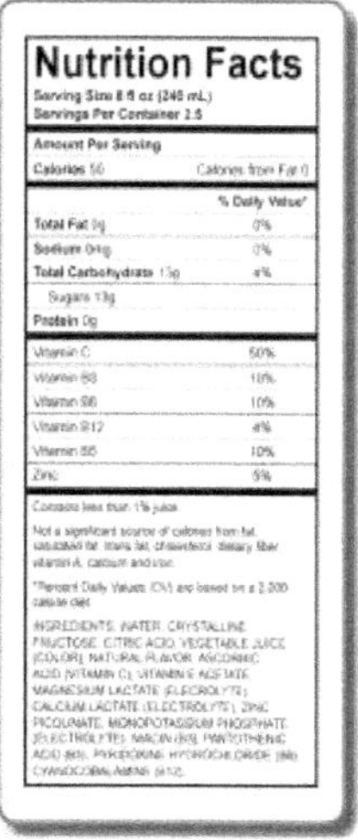

Calories from Beverages

- <u>Sweetened beverages</u>

- <u>Alcohol</u>

Beverage Choices without Calories

- Diet soda pop
- Tea* and Coffee*
- Water

*Plain – No added-sugar, creamer, etc...

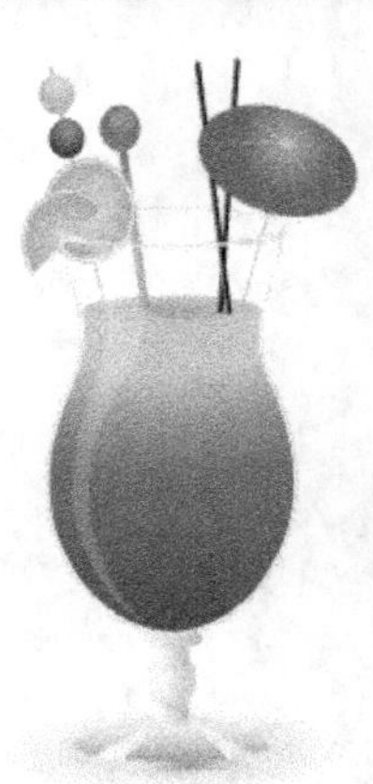

Portion sizes

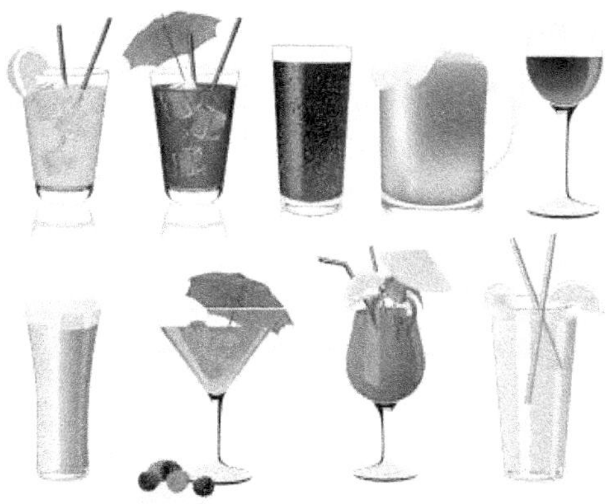

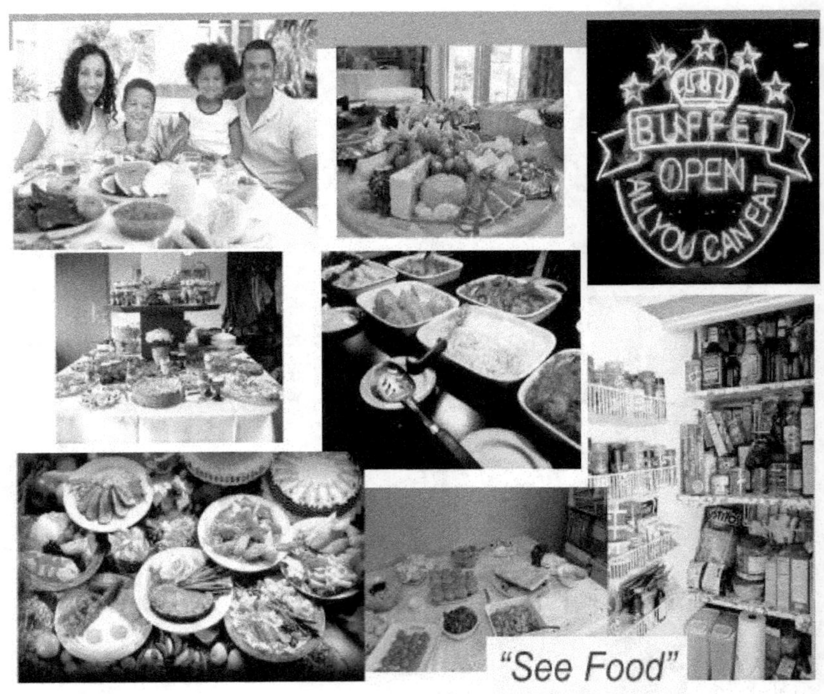

"See Food"

Ways to navigate the "buffet"

- Use a smaller plate

- Survey the options

- Limit choices to 3

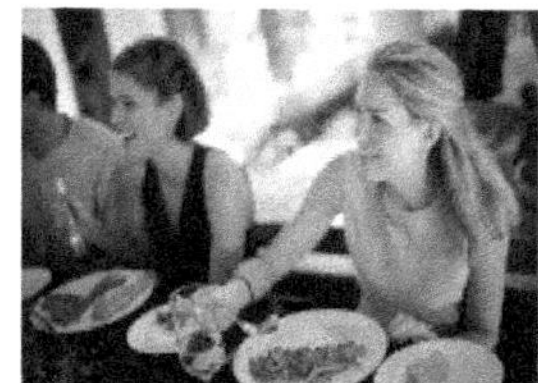

  - Aim for vegetables, legumes and fruit and less high calorie foods.

- Socialize away from the serving table

  - Conversation is calorie free

Remember your stomach can't count calories

New tastes = new hunger

What makes a website reliable?

Reliable	Caution
Look for	Chart rooms
- ".gov"	Discussion groups
- ".edu"	Personal stories
- ".org"	Quick fix solutions
Qualified Health Care Providers	Personal information
- MD, RN etc.	
Scientific references	
Contact information	
Recent content	

Examples of reliable websites

- http://www.eatright.org/
  - Information on food and nutrition. From the Academy of Nutrition and Dietetics (AND).
- http://www.choosemyplate.gov/
  - Information on food and nutrition. From the United States Department of Agriculture. (USDA)
- http://www.extension.umn.edu/
  - Information on creating a stronger Minnesota through education and research. University of Minnesota.
- http://www.mayoclinic.org/
  - Information on health conditions and nutrition. Mayo Clinic.

Summary

- Remember to read the nutrition facts label
  - Identify added sugars
  - Portions
  - Calories
- Be mindful of the "buffet effect"
- Use reliable internet resources

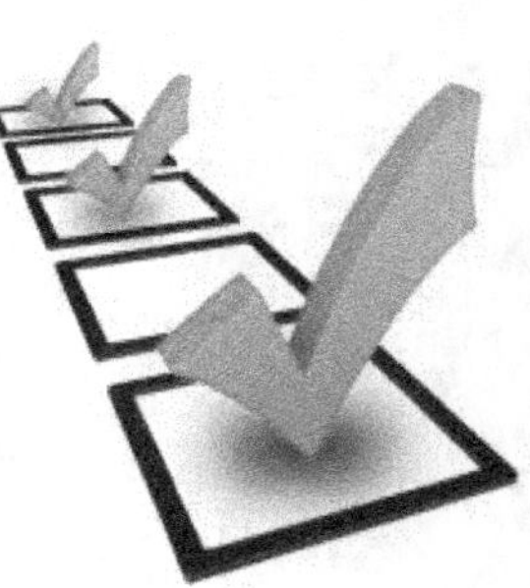

Resources

- "Added Sugars: Don't get Sabotaged by Sweeteners ." Mayo Foundation for Medical Education and Research. Web. Feb. 2016. http://www.mayoclinic.org/healthy-lifestyle/nutrition-and-healthy-eating/in-depth/added-sugar/art-20045328?pg=1.

- Hensrud, M.D., Donald. *The Mayo Clinic Diet Book*. Intercourse, PA: Good Books, 2010. Print.

- Online Health Information: What can you trust? National Institute of Health: U.S. National Library of Medicine. Web June 9. 2016.
https://www.nlm.nih.gov/medlineplus/ency/patientinstructions/000869.htm

- Rethink your Drink. Center for Disease Control and Prevention. Web Feb. 2016.
http://www.cdc.gov/healthyweight/healthy_eating/drinks.html.

- Rethinking your Drinking: Alcohol and your Health. U.S. Department of Health and Human Services. Web June. 2016. http://rethinkingdrinking.niaaa.nih.gov/tools/Calculators/calorie-calculator.aspx.